POCKET GUIDE FOR INTERNATIONAL DIETETICS AND NUTRITION TERMINOLOGY (IDNT) REFERENCE MANUAL:

Standardized Language for the Nutrition Care Process

First Edition

POCKET GUIDE FOR INTERNATIONAL DIETETICS AND
NUTRITION TERMINOLOGY (IDNT) REFERENCE MANUAL:
Standardized Language for the Nutrition Care Process
First Edition

ISBN: 978-0-88091-418-5

The views expressed in this publication are those of the authors and do not necessarily reflect policies and/or official positions of the American Dietetic Association. Mention of product names in this publication does not constitute endorsement by the authors or the American Dietetic Association. The American Dietetic Association disclaims responsibility for the application of the information contained herein.

10 9 8 7 6 5 4 3 2 1

Edition: 2008

POCKET GUIDE FOR INTERNATIONAL DIETETICS
AND NUTRITION TERMINOLOGY (IDNT) REFERENCE MANUAL:

Standardized Language for the Nutrition Care Process

First Edition

TABLE OF CONTENTS

ASSESSMENT

DIAGNOSIS

INTERVENTION

MONITOR & EVAL

Suggested references for diagnosis, intervention and monitoring and evaluation terms are
available in the *International Dietetics and Nutrition Terminology (IDNT) Reference Manual.*

Edition: 2008

Edition: 2008

Nutrition Care Process Summary

INTRODUCTION

Continually emerging from the American Dietetic Association's (ADA) strategic plan are priority actions that guide work groups and taskforces in creating tools to advance the dietetics profession. In 2002, to achieve the Association's strategic goals of promoting demand for dietetics practitioners and help them be more competitive in the marketplace, the ADA Quality Management Committee appointed the Nutrition Care Model Workgroup. This Workgroup developed the Nutrition Care Process and Model, a systematic process describing how dietetics practitioners provide care with patients/clients (1).

The nutrition care process is designed to improve the consistency and quality of individualized patient/client care and the predictability of the patient/client outcomes. It is not intended to standardize nutrition care for each patient/client but to establish a standardized process for providing care.

> **Special Note.** The terms **patient/client** are used in association with the NCP; however, the process is also intended for use with groups. In addition, family members or caregivers are an essential asset to the patient/client and dietetic practitioner in the NCP. Therefore, **groups, families, and caregivers** of patients/clients are implied each time a reference is made to patient/client.

There are four steps in the process—Nutrition Assessment, Nutrition Diagnosis, Nutrition Intervention, and Nutrition Monitoring and Evaluation. Three of the nutrition care process steps are very familiar to dietetics practitioners and nutrition textbooks skillfully cover their content—nutrition assessment, nutrition intervention, and nutrition monitoring and evaluation. However, the Workgroup identified a less well-defined aspect of nutrition care: nutrition diagnosis. Further, it recognized that a standard taxonomy for the second step in the process would greatly enhance the profession's ability to document, communicate, and research its impact.

As a result, the ADA's Standardized Language Task Force was formed to create a taxonomy for the profession's unique nutrition diagnosis language. The language was described during presentations at the 2005 Food and Nutrition Conference and Exhibition and made available in a publication at that meeting (2). The follow-up publication, *Nutrition Diagnosis and Intervention: Standardized Language for the Nutrition Care Process*, was published in 2007 (3). The nutrition diagnosis language is undergoing study in a number of research projects. This publication incorporates the first substantive changes to the nutrition diagnosis terminology. Future modifications will be made based on the results of the additional research.

The Standardized Language Task Force has examined in depth three of the four steps and developed and published standardized languages for: nutrition diagnosis, nutrition intervention, and now nutrition monitoring and evaluation. Through the committee's exploration of nutrition monitoring and evaluation, it is clear that there is substantial overlap between nutrition assessment and nutrition monitoring and evaluation. Many data points may be the same or related; however, the data purpose and use are distinct

1

in these two steps. We anticipate needing to add terms for Nutrition Assessment that are necessary to diagnose a nutrition problem, but would not be used for evaluating the impact of the nutrition intervention in the nutrition monitoring and evaluation step. Therefore, this publication illustrates a nearly complete language for describing the nutrition care process for nutrition practitioners and provides tools for practitioners to implement the process into their practice.

NUTRITION CARE PROCESS STEPS

Step 1. Nutrition Assessment

Nutrition assessment is the first step in the process and is a method for obtaining, verifying, and interpreting data that is needed to identify a nutrition-related problem. From the nutrition assessment data, the dietetic practitioner is able to determine whether a nutrition diagnosis/problem exists. This step, while well known to dietetics practitioners, would be greatly enhanced by use of standardized nutrition assessment language for communicating about patients/clients with similar disorders.

More effective comparison of nutrition assessment findings would be achieved with a standardized language. Thus, the Standardized Language Task Force will focus its efforts to describe the differences between nutrition assessment and nutrition monitoring and evaluation, which will be published in the future. Many opportunities for research exist in nutrition assessment, which will result in improved determinations of the most appropriate nutrition assessment data to use for individuals and populations and practice settings.

Step 2: Nutrition Diagnosis

Nutrition diagnosis is a critical step between nutrition assessment and nutrition intervention. The purpose of a standardized nutrition diagnosis language is to describe consistently nutrition problems so that they are clear within and outside the profession. The standard language will enhance communication and documentation of nutrition care, and it will provide a minimum data set and common data elements for future research.

In simple terms, a nutrition practitioner identifies and labels a specific nutrition diagnosis (problem) that, in general, he or she is responsible for treating independently (e.g., excessive carbohydrate intake). With nutrition intervention, the nutrition diagnosis ideally resolves, **or at least the signs and symptoms improve**. In contrast, a medical diagnosis describes a disease or pathology of organs or body systems (e.g., diabetes). In some instances, such as the nutrition diagnosis Swallowing Difficulty NC-1.1, nutrition practitioners are labeling or diagnosing the functional problem that has a nutritional consequence. Nutrition practitioners do not identify medical diagnoses; they diagnose phenomena in the nutrition domain.

ADA's Standardized Language Task Force developed a framework that outlines three domains—Clinical, Intake, and Behavioral-Environmental—within which the nutrition diagnoses/problems fall. With the changes incorporated from the research studies and recommendations accepted by the Task Force, sixty nutrition diagnoses/ problems have been identified. A reference was developed and it describes each nutrition diagnosis and incorporates expert input (2).

It is this step in the nutrition care process that results in the documentation of the nutrition diagnosis statement or PES statement. This statement is composed of three distinct components: the problem (P), the etiology (E) and the signs and symptoms (S). The PES statement is derived from the synthesis of information from the nutrition assessment data.

Step 3: Nutrition Intervention

Nutrition intervention is the third step in the nutrition care process. Nutrition interventions are specific actions used to remedy a nutrition diagnosis/problem, and can be used with individuals, a group, or the community at large. These nutrition interventions are intended to change a nutrition-related behavior, environmental condition, or aspect of nutritional health. A dietetics practitioner collaborates, whenever possible, with the patient/client(s) and other health care providers during the nutrition intervention.

Nutrition intervention consists of two interrelated components—planning and implementation. Planning involves prioritizing the nutrition diagnoses; conferring with the patient, others, and practice guides and policies; jointly establishing goals; and defining the nutrition prescription and identifying specific nutrition intervention(s). Implementing the nutrition intervention is the action phase, which includes carrying out and communicating the plan of care, continuing the data collection, and revising the nutrition intervention, as warranted, based on the patient/client response. This step cannot be completed unless both components are in place to support the nutrition intervention.

The nutrition intervention is, almost always, aimed at the etiology (E) of the nutrition diagnosis/problem identified in the PES statement. In very specific instances, the nutrition intervention is directed at reducing the effects of the signs and symptoms (S) to reduce the signs and symptoms. Generally, the signs and symptoms form the basis for the next step in the nutrition care process: nutrition monitoring and evaluation (Step 4).

Four domains of nutrition intervention have been identified—Food and/or Nutrient Delivery, Nutrition Education, Nutrition Counseling, and Coordination of Care. The terminology is defined and reference sheets for each specific nutrition intervention are available for use by the profession. It is believed that the information necessary for medical record documentation, billing, and the description of the nutrition interventions for research are included in the terminology.

A dietetics practitioner will note that while some interventions are closely related (e.g., education and counseling), the terms are intentionally separated to distinguish between them. Additionally, specific descriptors of a nutrition intervention encounter (i.e., interactions, visits, contacts, sessions) are provided to assist a dietetics practitioner with the details of his/her encounters with patient/client(s). Examples of descriptors include encounters with individuals or groups, face to face or electronically, and the degree to which the dietetics practitioner is responsible for the patient/client care, to name a few.

Edition: 2008

Step 4: Nutrition Monitoring and Evaluation

The purpose of nutrition monitoring and evaluation is to determine the amount of progress made by the patient/client and if goals are being met. Nutrition monitoring and evaluation tracks patient/client outcomes relevant to the nutrition diagnosis and intervention plans and goals. Nutrition care outcomes—the desired results of nutrition care—have been defined, and specific indicators that can be measured and compared to established criteria have been identified.

Selecting the appropriate nutrition care indicators is determined by the nutrition diagnosis and its etiology and signs or symptoms and the nutrition intervention used. The medical diagnosis and health care outcome goals, and quality management goals for nutrition also influence which nutrition care outcome indicators are chosen. Other factors, such as practice setting, patient/client population, and disease state and/or severity also affect the indicator selection.

The nutrition monitoring and evaluation outcomes are organized in four domains: Nutrition-Related Behavioral and Environmental Outcomes, Food and Nutrient Intake Outcomes, Nutrition-Related Physical Sign and Symptom Outcomes, and Nutrition-Related Patient/Client-Centered Outcomes.

During this step, dietetics practitioners monitor the patient/client progress by determining whether the nutrition intervention is being implemented and by providing evidence that the nutrition intervention is or is not *changing* the patient/client behavior or nutrition/health status. Dietetics practitioners measure the outcomes by selecting the appropriate nutrition care outcome indicator(s) and comparing the findings with previous status, nutrition intervention goals, and/or reference standards. The use of standardized indicators and criteria increases the validity and reliability of the outcome data and their collection facilitates electronic charting, coding, and outcomes measurement.

NUTRITION CARE PROCESS AND MEDICAL NUTRITION THERAPY

The nutrition care process and medical nutrition therapy (MNT) are not synonymous terms. MNT is one type of nutrition care, whereas the nutrition care process describes the approach to a spectrum of nutrition care. The nutrition care process defines specific steps a dietetics practitioner uses when providing MNT. Other activities, such as referral to a community program, are not MNT, but use the same nutrition care process.

IMPLEMENTATION OF THE NUTRITION CARE PROCESS AND FUTURE DIRECTIONS

Publications and Resources

The *International Dietetics and Nutrition Terminology Refernce Manual* represents the third major publication related to the nutrition care process in three years. Several exciting research projects are ongoing, including pilot tests of individual steps as well as multiple steps in the nutrition care process, which will influence future publications of this reference manual.

Dietetics practitioners across the country are implementing the nutrition care process. The reference manual provides extensive detail and explanation about the standardized language for dietetics. For a portable resource with essential excerpts from the reference manual, the ADA has created a companion publication—*Pocket Guide for International Dietetics and Nutrition Terminology Reference Manual, First Edition*.

At this time, three *Toolkits* are available from ADA for the on-line Evidence-Based Nutrition Practice Guidelines, based upon evidence analyses (4-6). They contain sample forms and examples incorporating the terms in the nutrition care process steps. These are available for purchase from ADA for dietetic practitioners to use at the "Store" tab at www.adaevidencelibrary.com. Dietetics practitioners may find useful the extensive resources provided on the ADA Web site, www.eatright.org, in the either the Research or Practice sections.

Members have completed numerous presentations and newsletter articles for national, state, and Dietetic Practice Group audiences, with nearly 8,000 individuals reached through presentations thus far. ADA also facilitates a peer network of dietetics practitioners who are leading the way in implementing the nutrition care process in their facilities and communities.

ADA is moving ahead in a variety of ways to implement the standardized language of the nutrition care process. In addition to numerous association activities, there are applications in the broader dietetics and medical communities.

International Information Sharing and Standardized Medical Languages

In 2005, the ADA Foundation funded an ADA hosted meeting to expand the dialogue with other international dietetic associations about ADA's standardized nutrition diagnosis language and similar efforts other associations have made. The meeting also initiated a dialogue between the foremost medical informatics organizations and the international nutrition and dietetics community. As a result of this dialogue:

- A presentation regarding the nutrition care process has been accepted at the XV International Congress of Dietetics, September 8 – 11, 2008 in Yokohama, Japan.

- The Dietitians Association of Australia has initiated a research study evaluating the face validity of the Nutrition Diagnoses.

- The Dutch Association of Dietitians (Nederlandse Vereniging van Diëtisten) has requested permission to use the Nutrition Diagnoses in their health care databases.

Indeed, as the world moves fully into electronic health care records, health informatics, and common databases, the international community of nutrition and dietetics practitioners have the opportunity to work in partnership with the medical informatics organizations to ensure that data elements critical to capturing nutrition care are included in databases and collected in a consistent way.

ADA is working toward including the concepts from the nutrition care process and the specific terms in standards for electronic health records and incorporation into standardized informatics languages, such as the Systematized Nomenclature of Medicine International (SNOMED), Logical Observation Identifiers Names and Codes (LOINC), and United Medical Language System (UMLS). ADA has already begun the dialogue with these groups to let them know the direction that the Association is headed and to keep them appraised of progress. Thus far, the feedback from the database and informatics groups has been quite positive, and they have expressed a need for documenting the unique nature of nutrition services.

SUMMARY

This publication contains all four steps in the nutrition care process, with a standardized taxonomy for nutrition diagnosis, nutrition intervention, and nutrition monitoring and evaluation. It represents the first revision to the nutrition diagnoses, enhanced information about nutrition counseling in the nutrition intervention section, and a new nutrition language for monitoring and evaluation. Various tools (e.g., reference sheets, patient/client examples, camera-ready pocket guides) are included for dietetics practitioners to implement the process in their practice. Future publications will provide a new taxonomy for nutrition assessment and revisions to the other steps based upon research findings.

From conception of the nutrition care process in 2002 through its implementation now, the Standardized Language Task Force continues to update ADA's House of Delegates, the Board of Directors, and members through reports, articles, presentations, publications, and the ADA Web site.

However, to see the strategic goals of an increased demand for dietetics practitioners who are more competitive in the marketplace come to fruition, practitioners need to take a historic step by implementing the nutrition care process today.

REFERENCES

1. Lacey K, Pritchett E. Nutrition care process and model: ADA adopts road map to quality care and outcomes management. *J Am Diet Assoc.* 2003;103:1061-1072.
2. American Dietetic Association. *Nutrition Diagnosis: A Critical Step in the Nutrition Care Process.* Chicago, IL: American Dietetic Association; 2006.
3. American Dietetic Association. *Nutrition Diagnosis and Intervention: Standardized Language for the Nutrition Care Process.* Chicago, IL: American Dietetic Association; 2007.
4. American Dietetic Association. Critical illness evidence-based nutrition guideline, 2006. Available at: http://www.adaevidencelibrary.com/topic.cfm?cat=2809. Accessed November 1, 2006.
5. American Dietetic Association. Disorders of Lipid Metabolism Toolkit. Available at: https://www.adaevidencelibrary.com/store.cfm. Accessed April 10, 2007.
6. American Dietetic Association. Adult Weight Management Evidence-Based Nutrition Practice Guideline, 2006. Available at: http://www.adaevidencelibrary.com/topic.cfm?cat=2798. Accessed April 10, 2007.

NCP Step 1. Nutrition Assessment

ASSESSMENT

What is the purpose of Nutrition Assessment? The purpose is to collect and interpret relevant patient/client* information to identify nutrition-related problems and their causes. This contrasts with nutrition monitoring and evaluation data where dietetics practitioners use similar, or even the same, data to determine changes in patient/client behavior or nutrition status and the efficacy of nutrition intervention.

How does a dietetics practitioner determine where to obtain Nutrition Assessment data? It depends on the practice setting. For individuals, data can come directly from the patient/client through interview, observation and measurements, in addition to information from the referring health care provider or agency, medical record and laboratory tests. For population groups, data from surveys, administrative data sets, and epidemiological or research studies are used. A nutrition assessment matrix that links nutrition assessment parameters with nutrition diagnoses was developed to assist practitioners in identifying nutrition diagnoses.

How are Nutrition Assessment data organized? In five categories.

> **Food/Nutrition History**—*Food and nutrient intake, nutrition related knowledge and practices, physical activity, and food availability*

> **Biochemical Data, Medical Tests, and Procedures**—*Laboratory data (e.g., electrolytes, glucose, lipid panel) and tests (e.g., gastric emptying time, resting metabolic rate)*

> **Anthropometric Measurements**—*Height, weight, body mass index, growth rate, and rate of weight change*

> **Physical Examination Findings**—*Oral health, physical appearance, muscle and subcutaneous fat, wasting, and mental status*

> **Client History**—*Medication and supplement use, medical/health history, and social, personal/family history*

What is done with the Nutrition Assessment data? Nutrition assessment data are compared to relevant norms and standards for interpretation and decision-making. These may be national, institutional, or regulatory norms and standards. Nutrition assessment findings are documented and are used in nutrition diagnosis statements and nutrition intervention goal setting.

Critical thinking during this step...
- Determining appropriate data to collect and selecting valid and reliable tools
- Distinguishing relevant from irrelevant data
- Selecting appropriate norms and standards for comparing the data
- Organizing and categorizing the data in a meaningful way that relates to nutrition problems

---

*Patient/client refers to individuals, groups, family members, and/or caregivers.

Edition: 2008

Is there a standardized language or taxonomy for Nutrition Assessment? Not at this time. Nutrition assessment has been well-described in the nutrition textbooks and literature. Use of standardized nutrition assessment procedures for patient/clients with similar disorders allows for effective comparison of nutrition assessment findings and outcome measurements resulting from nutrition intervention; therefore, the Nutrition Care Process Standardized Language Committee will articulate a nutrition assessment taxonomy to be published in a future edition.

Are dietetics practitioners limited to the Nutrition Assessment data included in the Nutrition Assessment Matrix and used in the Nutrition Diagnoses? Nutrition assessment data listed in the nutrition diagnoses reference sheets are undergoing study and research to confirm (validate) which data are most relevant to specific nutrition diagnoses. However, based on their patient/client population, practice setting and purpose, dietetics practitioners may utilize additional nutrition assessment parameters.

Detailed information about this step can be found in the International Dietetics and Nutrition Terminology (IDNT) Reference Manual: Standardized Language for the Nutrition Care Process, First Edition, American Dietetic Association.

Nutrition Assessment Matrix

Food and Nutrition History Data and Related Nutrition Diagnostic Terminology

Parameter (not all-inclusive)	Nutrition Diagnostic Terminology		
Excess intake of			
Alcohol and/or binge drinking	NI 4.3	NC 3.4	
Amino acids (specify)	NI 5.7.3		
Bioactive substances	NI 4.2		
Convenience foods, pre-prepared meals, and foods prepared away from home	NI 2.2	NB 2.4	
Energy from energy dense or high fat foods/beverages	NI 1.5	NI 2.2	NI 2.4
PN or EN	NC 3.3		
Fat, foods prepared with added fat	NI 5.4	NI 5.6.2	NC 2.2
Fat from high-risk lipids (saturated fat, trans fat, cholesterol)	NI 5.6.2	NI 5.6.3	
Fiber	NI 5.4	NI 5.8.6	NC 2.2
Fluid	NI 3.2		
Foods without available vitamins	NI 5.9.1		
Fortified foods and supplements containing vitamins	NI 5.9.2		
Food in a defined time period	NB 1.5		
Iron	NI 5.5		
Manganese	NI 5.5		
Mercury	NB 3.1		
Minerals	NI 5.10.2		
Parenteral or enteral nutrition	NI 1.5		
Phosphorus	NI 5.4	NC 2.2	
Plant foods containing soluble fiber, β-glucan, or plant sterol and stanol esters	NI 4.2		
Protein	NI 4.2 NC 2.2	NI 5.4	NI 5.7.2
Sodium	NI 3.2 NC 2.2	NI 5.4	
Substances which interfere with digestion or absorption	NI 4.2		
Associated factors			
Binge eating patterns	NI 2.2		
Change in way clothes fit	NC 3.2		
Highly variable calorie intake	NI 2.2		
Lipid or dextrose infusions, peritoneal dialysis or other medical treatments that provide significant calories	NI 2.4		

ASSESSMENT

Edition: 2008

Nutrition Assessment Matrix
Food and Nutrition History Data and Related Nutrition Diagnostic Terminology

Parameter (not all-inclusive)	Nutrition Diagnostic Terminology		
Insufficient intake of			
Carbohydrate	NI 5.8.1		
Energy	NI 1.4	NI 2.1	NI 5.2
Fiber, soy protein, β-glucan, or plant sterol and stanol esters	NI 4.1	NI 5.8.5	
Fluid	NI 3.1		
Fat, essential fatty acids	NI 5.6.1		
Fat, monounsaturated, polyunsaturated, or omega-3 fatty acids	NI 5.6.3		
Food/supplements and nutrients	NI 5.1 NI 5.10.1 NB 3.2	NI 5.3 NC 1.2	NI 5.9.1 NB 2.4
Food or food from specific foods/ groups due to GI symptoms	NC 1.4	NC 2.1	
Minerals	NI 5.10.1	NC 2.2	
Vitamins	NI 5.9.1	NC 2.2	
Parenteral or enteral nutrition	NI 1.4	NI 2.3	
Protein	NI 2.1	NI 5.2	NI 5.7.1
Vitamin D intake/sunlight exposure	NI 5.9.1	NI 5.10.1	
Associated factors			
Anorexia	NI 2.1	NI 5.10.2	NC 2.2
Changes in appetite or taste	NI 2.1	NC 2.3	
Changes in recent food intake	NC 1.2	NC 3.2	NC 3.4
Failure to recognize foods	NB 2.6		
Forgets to eat	NB 2.6		
Hunger	NC 3.1	NB 3.2	
Infant coughing, crying, latching on and off, pounding on breasts	NC 1.3		
Infant lethargy	NC 1.3		
Infant with decreased feeding frequency/duration, early cessation of feeding, and/or feeding resistance	NC 1.3		
Infant with fewer than six wet diapers in 24 hours	NC 1.3		
Infant with hunger, lack of satiety after feeding	NC 1.3		
Lack of interest in food	NI 1.4 NI 5.10.1	NI 5.2	NI 5.9.1
Lack of strength or stamina for eating	NB 2.6		
Mealtime resistance	NC 1.1		
Mother doesn't hear infant swallowing	NC 1.3		
Mother with lack of confidence in ability to breastfeed	NC 1.3		
Mother with small amount of milk when pumping	NC 1.3		

Nutrition Assessment Matrix
Food and Nutrition History Data and Related Nutrition Diagnostic Terminology

Parameter (not all-inclusive)	Nutrition Diagnostic Terminology		
Associated factors, cont'd			
Nausea	NI 2.1	NC 2.2	
Recent food avoidance and or/lack of interest in food	NI 5.3		
Refusal to eat; chew	NC 3.1	NB 2.6	
Satiety, early	NC 3.2		
Spitting food out or prolonged feeding time	NC 1.2		
Swallowing, difficulty	NI 3.1		
Thirst	NI 3.1		
Intake different from recommended			
Carbohydrate	NI 5.8.2	NI 5.8.3	NI 5.8.4
Carbohydrate, protein and/or fat intake from enteral and/or parenteral nutrients	NI 2.5		
Food, inappropriate use of	NB 2.6		
Food choices, inappropriate	NI 5.8.1		
Food group/nutrient imbalance	NB 1.2		
Food intake includes raw eggs, unpasturized milk products, soft cheeses, undercooked meats, wild plants, berries and mushrooms	NB 3.1		
Food variety, limited	NB 3.2		
Intake that does not support replacement or mitigation of OTC, prescribed drugs, herbals, botanicals, or dietary supplements	NC 2.3		
Medication (over the counter or prescribed), herbal, botanical, or dietary supplement intake that is problematic or inconsistent with recommended foods	NC 2.3		
Protein or other supplementation	NI 5.7.2	NI 5.7.3	
US Dietary Guidelines, any nutrient	NI 5.9.2	NB 1.7	
Food and nutrient intolerance			
Allergic reactions to certain carbohydrate foods or food groups	NI 5.8.3		
Coughing and choking with eating	NC 1.1		
Decreased intake or avoidance of food difficult to form into a bolus	NC 1.2		
Diminished joint mobility or wrist, hand or digits that impair ability to independently consume food	NI 1.4	NI 5.8.1	
Diarrhea in response to high refined carbohydrate intake	NI 5.8.3		
Dropping cups, utensils	NB 2.6		

11

Nutrition Assessment Matrix
Food and Nutrition History Data and Related Nutrition Diagnostic Terminology

Parameter (not all-inclusive)	Nutrition Diagnostic Terminology	
Food and nutrient intolerance, cont'd		
Dropping food from utensil on repeated attempts to feed	NB 2.6	
Feeling of food "getting stuck" in throat	NC 1.1	
Foods provided not conducive to self feeding	NB 2.6	
Nausea, vomiting, diarrhea, high gastric residual volume	NI 2.5	
Pain on swallowing	NC 1.1	
Poor lip closure, drooling	NC 1.1	NB 2.6
Pouching food	NC 1.1	
Prolonged chewing, feeding time	NC 1.1	
Utensil biting	NB 2.6	
Nutrition and health awareness		
Avoidance of food or calorie containing beverages	NB 1.5	NC 1.1
Avoidance of foods of age-appropriate texture	NC 1.2	
Avoidance of foods/food groups	NB 1.2	
Belief that aging can be slowed by dietary limitations	NB 3.2	
Chronic dieting behavior	NI 5.10.1	NB 1.5
Cultural or religious practices that limit intake	NI 5.7.1	
Cultural or religious practices that limit modification of dietary carbohydrate intake	NI 5.8.2	
Defensiveness, hostility, or resistance to change	NB 1.3	
Denial of hunger	NB 1.5	
Denial of need for food- and nutrition-related changes	NB 1.3	
Eating alone, feeling embarrassed by the amount of food eaten	NB 1.5	
Eating much more rapidly than normal, eating until feeling uncomfortably full, consuming large amounts of food when not feeling hungry	NB 1.5	
Embarrassment or anger at need for self-monitoring	NB 1.4	NB 2.3
Emotional distress, anxiety, or frustration surrounding mealtimes	NB 2.6	

Nutrition Assessment Matrix
Food and Nutrition History Data and Related Nutrition Diagnostic Terminology

Parameter (not all-inclusive)	Nutrition Diagnostic Terminology		
Nutrition and health awareness, cont'd			
Excessive reliance on nutrition terming and preoccupation with nutrient content of food	NB 1.5		
Expected food/nutrition related outcomes are not achieved	NB 1.6		
Failure to complete any agreed homework	NB 1.6		
Failure to keep appointments/schedule or engage in counseling	NB 1.3	NB 1.6	
Fear of foods or dysfunctional thoughts regarding food or food experiences	NB 1.5		
Feeling disgusted with oneself, depressed, or guilty after overeating	NB 1.5		
Food faddism, pica	NC 3.1	NB 1.2	NB 3.2
Food preoccupation	NB 1.5		
Frustration or dissatisfaction with MNT recommendations	NB 2.5		
Frustration over lack of control	NB 2.5		
Harmful beliefs and attitudes of parent/ caregiver	NB 3.2		
Incomplete self-monitoring records	NB 1.4		
Inflexibility with food selection	NB 1.5		
Irrational thoughts about food's effect on the body	NB 1.5		
Knowledge about current fad diets	NB 1.5		
Lack of appreciation of the importance of making recommended nutrition-related changes	NB 1.6		
Negative body language (note: varies by culture)	NB 1.3		
Previous failures to effectively change target behavior	NB 1.3		
Prolonged use of substances known to increase vitamin requirements or reduce vitamin absorption	NI 5.9.1		
Sense of lack of control of overeating during the episode	NB 1.5		
Unwillingness or disinterest in applying nutrition related recommendations	NC 3.3		
Verbalizes unwillingness/disinterest in learning	NB 1.1		
Weight preoccupation	NB 1.5		

Edition: 2008

Nutrition Assessment Matrix
Food and Nutrition History Data and Related Nutrition Diagnostic Terminology

Parameter (not all-inclusive)	Nutrition Diagnostic Terminology	
Food and nutrient knowledge and skill		
Food and nutrition-related knowledge deficit	NI 5.1	NC 2.2
Inability to apply food- and nutrition-related information	NC 3.3	NB 1.1
Inability to apply guideline information	NB 1.7	
Inability to change food- or activity-related behavior	NB 2.5	
Inability to interpret data or self management tools	NB 2.3	
Inability to maintain weight or regain of weight	NC 3.3	
Inability to recall agreed upon changes	NB 1.6	
Inability or unwillingness to select, or disinterest in selecting food consistent with guidelines	NB 1.7	
Inaccurate or incomplete understanding of information related to guidelines or needed changes	NB 1.1	NB 1.7
Lack of ability to prepare meals	NI 5.3	
Lack of compliance or inconsistent compliance with plan	NB 1.6	
Lack of efficacy to make changes or to overcome barriers to change	NB 1.3	
Limited knowledge of carbohydrate composition of foods or of carbohydrate metabolism	NI 5.8.3	
Mother has insufficient knowledge of breastfeeding or infant hunger/satiety signals	NC 1.3	
Mother is concerned about breastfeeding/ lack of support	NC 1.3	
No prior knowledge of need for food and nutrition-related recommendations	NB 1.1	
Provides inaccurate or incomplete written response to questionnaire/written tool, or is unable to read written tool	NB 1.1	
Relates concerns about previous attempts to learn information	NB 1.1	NB 2.5
Uncertainty as to how to consistently apply food/nutrition information	NB 1.6	
Uncertainty of how to complete monitoring records	NB 1.4	

Nutrition Assessment Matrix
Food and Nutrition History Data and Related Nutrition Diagnostic Terminology

Parameter (not all-inclusive)	Nutrition Diagnostic Terminology		
Food and nutrient knowledge and skill, cont'd			
Uncertainty regarding appropriate foods to prepare based upon nutrition prescription	NB 2.4		
Uncertainty regarding changes that could/ should be made in response to data in self-monitoring records	NB 1.4	NB 2.3	
Uncertainty regarding nutrition-related recommendations	NC 3.3		
Physical activity			
Decreased or sedentary activity level (due to barriers or other reasons)	NC 3.3		
Increased physical activity	NI 1.2	NC 3.1	NB 2.2
Excessive physical activity (ignoring family, job; exercising without rest/ rehabilitation days, or while injured or sick)	NB 1.5	NB 2.2	
Low level of NEAT (non-exercise activity thermogenesis)	NB 2.1		
Overtraining	NB 2.2		
Food availability			
Economic constraints that limit availability of appropriate foods	NI 2.1 NI 5.8.4	NI 5.8.2	NI 5.8.3
Food insecurity/unwillingness to use available resources	NB 2.5		
Inability to purchase and transport foods to one's home	NB 2.4		
Intake consistent with estimated or measured energy needs	NC 3.4		
Lack of facilities or accommodations for breastfeeding in community or at work	NC 1.3		
Ready access to available foods/products with bioactive substance	NI 4.2		
Unfavorable QOL or other quality of life rating	NB 2.5		
Other			
Ethnic and cultural related issues	NB 2.5		
Extreme hunger with or without palpitations, tremor, sweating	NC 3.4		
Lack of social and familial support	NB 2.5		
Intake consistent with estimated or measured energy needs	NC 3.4		
No self-management equipment	NB 1.4		
Normal intake in the face of illness	NC 3.2		
Use of narcotics	NC 3.4		

Updated: 2008 Edition

Nutrition Assessment Matrix
Anthropometric Data and Related Nutrition Diagnostic Terminology

Parameter (not all-inclusive)	Findings	Nutrition Diagnostic Terminology		
Anthropometric Data				
Body Mass Index (BMI)	decreased	NI 2.3	NI 5.1	NI 5.2
		NC 3.1	NB 1.5	NB 3.2
BMI	increased	NI 1.5	NC 3.3	NB 1.5
		NB 2.1		
Body fat distribution	changed	NC 3.4		
Body fat percentage	increased	NI 1.5		
Growth	delayed	NI 1.2	NI 2.1	NI 2.3
		NI 5.1	NI 5.2	NI 5.3
		NI 5.5	NI 5.7.2	NI 5.9.2
		NC 2.1	NB 1.4	NB 2.2
		NB 3.2		
Height	loss	NI 5.10.1		
Muscle circumference, mid-arm	decreased	NI 5.1	NC 3.1	
Muscle mass	increased	NI 1.2		
Skinfold thickness	increased	NC 3.3		
Skinfold thickness	decreased	NI 5.1	NC 3.1	
Waist circumference	increased	NC 3.3		
Wasting		NI-5.2		
Weight	change, rapid	NC 2.2	NB 1.5	
Weight	loss	NI 1.4	NI 2.1	NI 2.3
		NI 2.5	NI 3.1	NI 4.2
		NI 5.2	NI 5.3	NI 5.6.1
		NC 1.3	NC 2.1	NC 3.2
		NB 2.2	NB 2.6	
	unintentional	NI 1.2	NI 5.1	NI 5.2
		NI 2.3		
Weight	decreased	NC 3.1	NB 2.2	
Weight	gain	NI 1.4	NI 1.5	NI 2.2
		NI 3.2	NC 2.3	NC 3.3
		NC 3.4		
	in excess of lean tissue accretion	NI 2.4	NI 2.5	
	interdialytic	NI 5.4		
Weight	failure to gain as planned	NI 2.3	NI 5.2	NI 5.3
		NC 1.3	NB 1.6	NB 2.2

Updated: 2008 Edition

Nutrition Assessment Matrix
Biochemical Data, Medical Tests, and Procedures and Related Nutrition Diagnostic Terminology

Parameter (not all-inclusive)	Findings	Nutrition Diagnostic Terminology		
Biochemical data				
3-methyl histidine, urine	increased	NI 5.7.3		
Albumin, serum	decreased	NI 5.1	NI 5.2	NC 3.4
Alcohol, blood	increased	NI 4.3		
Alpha tocopherol, plasma	decreased	NI 5.9.1		
Amino acids (specific levels)	increased	NI 5.7.3	NC 2.1	
Ammonia, serum	increased	NI 5.7.3	NC 2.2	
Amylase, serum	increased	NI 5.6.2	NI 5.6.3	
AST, aspartate aminotransferase	increased	NI 4.3	NC 2.2	NB 2.2
ALT, alanine aminotransferase	increased	NC 2.2		
Bilirubin, total serum	increased	NI 5.6.2	NI 5.6.3	NC 2.2
BUN	increased	NI 3.1	NI 5.4	NI 5.7.2
BUN:creatinine ratio	increased	NI 5.7.3 NB 1.5	NI 2.4	NC 2.2
Calcium, serum	decreased	NI 2.3		
Calcium, serum ionized	decreased	NI 5.9.1		
Calcium, serum ionized	increased	NI 5.9.2		
Calcium, urine	decreased	NI 5.10.1		
Chloride, serum	decreased	NB 1.5		
Cholesterol, HDL	decreased	NI 5.4 NI 5.10.2	NI 5.6.2	NI 5.6.3
Cholesterol, LDL	increased	NI 5.4	NI 5.6.2	NI 5.6.3
Cholesterol, serum	decreased	NI 4.2	NI 5.1	
Cholesterol, serum	increased	NI 5.4 NB 1.5	NI 5.6.2	NI 5.6.3
Copper	decreased	NI 2.3	NI 5.10.1	
Cortisol levels	increased	NB 2.2		
C-reactive protein	elevated	NI 5.1	NI 5.6.3	
Creatinine	elevated	NI 5.4	NC 2.2	
Digestive enzymes	altered	NC 1.4	NC 2.1	
D-xylose	abnormal	NC 1.4	NC 2.1	
Fat, fecal	increased	NI 5.6.2	NC 1.4	NC 2.1
Ferritin, serum	decreased	NB 2.2		
Ferritin, serum	increased	NI 5.10.2		
Folic acid, serum	decreased	NI 5.9.1		
Folic acid, erythrocyte		NI 5.9.2		
GFR, glomerular filtration rate	decreased	NI 5.4 NC 2.2	NI 5.7.2	NI 5.7.3
GGT, gamma-glutamyl transferase	elevated	NI 4.3		

17

Edition: 2008

ASSESSMENT

Nutrition Assessment Matrix
Biochemical Data, Medical Tests, and Procedures and Related Nutrition Diagnostic Terminology

Parameter (not all-inclusive)	Findings	Nutrition Diagnostic Terminology		
Biochemical data, cont'd				
Glucose, blood	increased	NI 2.4 NI 5.8.4	NI 5.8.2 NC 2.2	NI 5.8.3 NC 3.4
Glucose, blood	decreased	NI 5.8.3 NB 1.5	NI 5.8.4	NC 2.2
Glucose, blood	inadequate control	NC 2.2		
Glutathione reductase, erythrocyte	increased	NI 5.9.1		
GTT (glucose tolerance test)	abnormal	NI 5.8.2		
Hematocrit	increased	NB 2.2		
Hemoglobin	decreased	NI 5.10.1		
Hemoglobin A1c	increased	NI 5.8.2	NC 2.2	
Hormone levels	fluctuating	NC 3.4		
Homocysteine	increased	NI 5.9.1		
Hydrogen breath test	abnormal	NC 1.4	NC 2.1	
IGF binding protein	abnormal	NB 2.2		
Immune function	suppressed	NB 2.2		
Iodine, urinary	decreased	NI 5.10.1		
Iron	decreased	NI 2.3		
Iron binding capacity	decreased	NI 2.3		
Ketones, urine	present	NB 1.5		
Leucopenia	present	NB 1.5		
Lipase	increased	NI 5.6.2	NI 5.6.3	
Lipid profile, serum	abnormal	NC 2.2 NB 1.7	NC 3.4	NB 1.5
Liver enzymes	elevated	NI 1.5 NI 4.2 NI 5.6.3	NI 2.4 NI 5.4 NC 2.2	NI 2.5 NI 5.6.2 NB 2.2
Magnesium, serum	decreased	NI 5.1	NI 5.5	NI 5.10.1
Magnesium, serum	increased	NI 5.10.2		
Mean corpuscular volume	increased	NI 4.3		
N'methyl-nicotanimide	decreased	NI 5.9.1		
N'methyl-nicotanimide	increased	NI 5.9.2		
Osmolality, serum	increased	NI 3.1		
Osmolality, serum	decreased	NI 3.2		
Parathyroid hormone	increased	NI 5.9.1	NI 5.9.2	
pCO$_2$	abnormal	NI 2.4	NC 2.2	
Phosphorus, serum	decreased	NI 5.1 NI 5.10.1	NI 5.5	NI 5.9.1
Phosphorus, serum	increased	NI 2.5	NI 5.4	NI 5.10.2
pO$_2$	abnormal	NC 2.2		

Edition: 2008   18

Nutrition Assessment Matrix
Biochemical Data, Medical Tests, and Procedures and Related Nutrition Diagnostic Terminology

Parameter (not all-inclusive)	Findings	Nutrition Diagnostic Terminology		
Biochemical data, cont'd				
Potassium, serum	decreased	NI 2.5 NC 2.2	NI 5.1 NB 1.5	NI 5.5
Potassium, serum	increased	NI 5.1	NI 5.4	NC 2.2
Prealbumin	decreased	NI 5.1		
Pyrodoxal 5'phosphate, plasma	decreased	NI 5.9.1		
Pyrodoxal 5'phosphate, plasma	increased	NI 5.9.2		
Retinol, serum	decreased	NI 5.9.1		
Retinol, serum	increased	NI 5.9.2		
Sodium, serum	decreased	NI 3.2	NC 3.4	NB 1.5
Sodium, serum	increased	NI 3.1		
Stool culture	positive	NC 1.4	NB 3.1	
Thyroid function tests (TSH, T4, T3)	abnormal	NI 5.10.2	NB 1.5	
Toxicology reports	positive	NB 3.2		
Transketolase activity, erythrocyte	increased	NI 5.9.1		
Transferrin	increased	NI 4.3		
Triene:tetraene ratio	increased	NI 5.6.1		
Triglycerides	increased	NI 5.4	NI 5.6.2	NI 5.6.3
Vitamin B12	decreased	NI 5.9.1		
Vitamin C, plasma	decreased	NI 5.9.1		
Vitamin K (PT, PTT, INR)	abnormal	NI 2.3	NI 5.9.1	NI 5.9.2
Zinc, serum	decreased	NI 2.3	NB 2.2	
Medical tests and procedures				
Gastric emptying study	abnormal	NC 1.4		
Mineral density, bone	decreased	NI 5.10.1		
Respiratory quotient	abnormal	NI 1.5	NI 2.3	
Metabolic rate, resting	increased	NI 1.2		
Small bowel transit time	abnormal	NC 1.4		

Updated: 2008 Edition

Nutrition Assessment Matrix
Physical Examination Data and Related Nutrition Diagnostic Terminology

Parameter (not all-inclusive)	Findings	Nutrition Diagnostic Terminology		
Head and neck				
Eyes:				
Bitot's spots	present	NI 5.9.1		
Dryness	present	NI 5.9.2		
Night blindness	present	NI 5.9.1		
Vision	decreased	NC 3.2		
Xeropthalmia	present	NI 5.9.1		
Tongue:				
Bright red	present	NI 5.9.1		
Glossitis	present	NI 5.9.1	NC 2.1	
Extrusion	present	NB 2.6		
Impaired tongue movement	present	NC 1.2		
Frenulum abnormality (infants)	present	NC 1.3		
Magenta	present	NI 5.9.1		
Taste, sense	decreased	NC 3.2		
Mouth and throat:				
Cheilosis	present	NI 5.9.1	NC 2.1	
Dry mucous membranes, hoarse or wet voice, tongue extrusion	present	NI 2.3 NC 1.1 NB 3.1	NI 3.1 NC 1.2	NI 5.9.2 NB 2.6
Gums, inflamed or bleeding	present	NI 2.3	NI 5.1	NI 5.9.1
Ketone smell on breath	present	NI 5.8.1		
Lesions, oral	present	NC 1.2	NC 2.1	
Lips	dry or cracked	NI 5.9.2		
Mucosa (mouth and pharynx)	edema	NI 5.9.1		
Parotid glands	enlarged	NB 1.5		
Stomatitis	present	NI 5.9.1		
Teeth	missing, caries, damaged enamel, poorly fitting dentures	NI 1.4 NB 1.5	NI 5.8.2	NC 1.2
Head:				
Cranial nerve function (V, VII, IX, X, XII)	altered	NC 1.1	NC 1.2	
Fontanelle, bulging (in infants)	present	NI 5.9.2		
Hair, changes, brittle and lifeless	present	NI 5.10.2	NB 1.5	

Nutrition Assessment Matrix
Physical Examination Data and Related Nutrition Diagnostic Terminology

Parameter (not all-inclusive)	Findings	Nutrition Diagnostic Terminology		
Head, cont'd:				
Hairs, coiled	present	NI 5.9.1		
Hair loss	present	NI 2.3 NI 5.9.2	NI 5.1	NI 5.2
Headache	present	NI 5.9.2		
Lanugo hair formation on face and trunk	present	NB 1.5		
Mucosa, nasal	dryness	NI 5.9.2		
Occipital wasting	present	NI 5.2		
Smell, sense	decreased	NC 3.2		
Gastrointestinal system				
Ascites	present	NI 3.2	NC 2.2	
Bowel sounds	abnormal	NC 1.4	NC 2.1	
Constipation	present	NI 4.2	NI 5.5	NC 1.4
Distention, abdominal	present	NC 1.4	NC 2.1	
Diarrhea	present	NI 2.3	NI 4.2	NI 5.5
Diarrhea in response to carbohydrate feeding	present	NI 5.8.2		
Nausea	present	NI 2.3	NI 5.9.2	
Vomiting	present	NI 2.3	NI 5.9.2	
Neurologic system				
Confusion	present	NI 5.9.1		
Concentration	impaired	NB 1.5		
Motor and gait disturbances	present	NI 5.9.1		
Neurological changes	present	NI 4.2	NI 5.7.3	
Vibratory and position sense	decreased	NI 5.9.1		
Cardiovascular-pulmonary system				
Cardiovascular changes	arrythmias	NI 4.2	NB 1.5	
Edema, pulmonary	crackles or rales	NI 3.2		

Edition: 2008

Nutrition Assessment Matrix
Physical Examination Data and Related Nutrition Diagnostic Terminology

Parameter (not all-inclusive)	Findings	Nutrition Diagnostic Terminology		
Extremities and musculoskeletal system				
Arthralgia; joint effusions	present	NI 5.9.1		
Bone alterations	fragility	NI 5.9.2		
Bones	obvious prominence	NI 5.2		
Bones, long	widening at ends	NI 5.9.1		
Fat, body	decreased	NC 3.2 NB 2.2	NC 3.3	NB 1.5
Fat, body	increased	NC 3.3	NB 3.2	
Hands and feet	cyanosis	NB 1.5		
Hands and feet	tingling and numbness	NI 5.9.1		
Injuries	frequent and prolonged	NB 2.2		
Muscle mass	decreased	NI 2.3 NB 1.5	NI 2.5 NB 2.1	NI 5.1
Muscle soreness	chronic	NB 2.2		
Nail beds	blue, clubbing	NC 2.2		
Nail beds	pale	NI 2.3	NI 5.1	
Nail changes	present	NI 5.10.2		
Russell's sign	present	NB 1.5		
Skin				
Calcification of soft tissues (calcinosis)	present	NI 5.9.2		
Changes consistent with nutrient deficiency/excess	present	NI 5.6.1	NB 1.7	NB 3.2
Dermatitis	present	NI 5.6.1	NI 5.6.3	
Edema, peripheral	present	NI 2.4 NC 2.2	NI 2.5 NB 1.5	NI 5.2
Erythema, scaling and peeling of the skin	present	NI 5.9.2		
Ecchymosis	present	NI 5.9.1		
Follicular hyperkeratosis	present	NI 5.9.1		
Jaundice and itching	present	NC 2.2		
Skin	dry, scaly	NI 2.1 NI 5.6.1	NI 3.1 NB 1.5	NI 5.2
Skin integrity	decreased	NI 2.3	NI 5.1	
Skin lesions	present	NI 5.9.1		
Skin turgor	decreased	NI 3.1	NC 1.1	

Nutrition Assessment Matrix
Physical Examination Data and Related Nutrition Diagnostic Terminology

Parameter (not all-inclusive)	Findings	Nutrition Diagnostic Terminology		
Skin, cont'd				
Skin turgor	increased	NI 2.3	NI 3.2	NI 5.4
Seborrheic dermatitis	present	NI 5.9.1		
Perifolicular hemorrhages	present	NI 5.9.1		
Petechiae	present	NI 5.9.1		
Pressure ulcers (stage II-IV)	present	NI 2.3	NI 5.1	
Wound healing	decreased	NI 5.1 NI 5.9.1	NI 5.2	NI 5.3
Xanthomas	present	NI 5.6.2	NI 5.6.3	
Vital signs				
Blood pressure	decreased	NI 5.2	NB 1.5	
Blood pressure	increased	NI 4.2		
Heart rate	decreased	NB 1.5		
Heart rate	increased	NC 3.2		
Respiratory rate	increased	NI 1.5	NC 3.2	
Temperature	decreased	NB 1.5		
Temperature	increased	NI 1.2	NC 3.2	
Urine output	decreased	NI 3.1		
Miscellaneous				
Body language (note: varies by culture)	negative	NB 1.3	NB 1.6	

Updated: 2008 Edition

Nutrition Assessment Matrix
Client History Data and Related Diagnostic Terminology

Parameter (not all-inclusive)	Nutrition Diagnostic Terminology		
Social history			
Abuse, physical, sexual or emotional	NC 3.3		
Alcohol intake during pregnancy despite knowledge of risk	NI 4.3		
Alcohol intake, excessive	NI 4.3	NC 1.2	
Avoidance of social events where food is served	NB 1.5		
Change in living environment/ independence	NI 5.10.1		
Chronic non-compliance	NB 1.3		
Substance abuse	NI 1.4	NC 3.2	NB 1.5
Environmental conditions, e.g., infants exclusively fed breast milk with limited exposure to sunlight (vitamin D)	NI 5.9.1		
Geographic latitude and history of UVB exposure/sunscreen use	NI 5.10.1		
Geographic location and socioeconomic status associated with altered nutrient intake of indigenous phenomenon	NI 5.2		
Giving birth to an infant with fetal alcohol syndrome	NI 4.3		
Hunger in the face of inadequate access to food supply	NI 5.3		
Illness or physical disability	NC 3.1	NB 3.2	
Lack of ability to prepare meals	NI 5.3		
Lack of developmental readiness	NC 1.2		
Lack of funds for purchase of appropriate foods	NI 5.3		
Lack of suitable support system to access food	NB 3.2		
Lifestyle changes, recent	NB 2.5		
Low cardiorespiratory fitness and/or low muscle strength	NB 2.1		
New medical diagnosis or change in existing diagnosis or condition	NI 4.3 / NB 2.3	NB 1.1 / NB 2.5	NB 1.4
Occupation of athlete, dancer, gymnast	NC 3.1		
Physical activity, easy fatigue with increased activity; unable to achieve desired levels	NI 2.3		
Physical disability or limitation	NC 3.3	NB 2.6	
Unrealistic expectations of weight gain or ideal weight	NI 2.4		
Personal/Family history			
Of childhood obesity	NC 3.3		
Of eating disorders, depression, obsessive compulsive disorders, anxiety disorders	NB 1.5		
Of familial obesity	NC 3.3		

Nutrition Assessment Matrix
Client History Data and Related Diagnostic Terminology

Parameter (not all-inclusive)	Nutrition Diagnostic Terminology		
Personal/Family history, cont'd			
Of hyperlipidemia, atherosclerosis, or pancreatitis	NI 5.6.2	NI 5.6.3	
Of inability to lose weight through conventional weight loss intervention	NC 3.3		
Medical/Health history			
AIDS/HIV	NI 2.1 NI 5.6.1	NI 2.3 NC 3.2	NI 5.1
Alcoholism	NI 1.4	NC 2.2	
Alzheimer's disease	NI 1.2 NB 2.6	NI 3.1	NC 1.2
Anemia	NI 5.6.1 NB 1.5	NI 5.9.1	NI 5.10.1
Anxiety disorder	NI 2.2	NB 2.1	
Arthritis	NB 2.1		
Asthma	NC 3.4		
Atherosclerosis	NI 5.6.2		
Biliary disease	NI 5.6.2	NI 5.6.3	
Binge eating	NB 2.2		
Breast surgery	NC 1.3		
Bulimia nervosa	NB 2.2		
Burns	NI 2.3	NI 5.1	NC 3.2
Cadidiasis	NC 1.3		
Cancer, head, neck or pharyngeal	NC 1.2		
Cancer (other)	NI 5.9.2	NC 3.2	NB 1.2
Cardiac, neurologic, respiratory changes	NB 3.1		
Cardiovascular disease	NI 3.2 NI 5.3 NI 5.9.2 NB 2.3	NI 4.1 NI 5.4 NC 2.2	NI 4.2 NI 5.6.3 NB 1.2
Celiac disease	NI 5.8.1 NC 1.4	NI 5.9.1 NC 2.1	NI 5.10.1
Cerebral palsy	NI 1.2	NC 1.2	NB 2.4
Chronic fatigue syndrome	NB 2.1		
Chronic obstructive pulmonary disease	NI 1.2	NC 3.2	
Chronic or acute disease or trauma, geographic location and socioeconomic status associated with nutrient intake of indigenous phenomenon	NI 5.2		
Cleft lip/palate	NC 1.2	NC 1.3	
Cognitive or emotional impairment	NB 2.3	NB 2.4	
Constipation	NI 5.8.5	NI 5.8.6	
Crohn's disease	NI 2.3 NC 1.4	NI 5.1 NC 2.1	
Cushing's syndrome	NC 3.4		
Cystic fibrosis	NI 1.2	NI 5.6.2	
Dementia	NI 1.2 NB 2.6	NI 1.4 NB 3.2	NI 3.1

Edition: 2008

Nutrition Assessment Matrix
Client History Data and Related Diagnostic Terminology

Parameter (not all-inclusive)	Nutrition Diagnostic Terminology		
Medical/Health history, cont'd			
Depression	NI 2.1	NI 4.3	NC 3.2
	NC 3.3	NB 1.5	NB 2.1
Developmental delay	NB 2.6		
Diabetes mellitus	NI 5.6.3	NI 5.8.2	NI 5.8.3
	NI 5.8.4	NC 2.2	NB 1.2
	NB 1.4	NB 2.3	
Diverticulitis	NI 5.8.6	NC 1.4	
Dysphasia	NC 1.1		
Eating disorder	NI 1.4	NI 5.8.6	
Encephalopathy, hepatic	NI 5.4		
Fatigue	NC 3.4		
Fluorosis	NI 5.10.2		
Foodborne illness, e.g., bacterial, viral, and parasitic infection	NB 3.1		
Fractures, stress	NB 2.2		
Gastrointestinal stricture	NI 5.8.6		
Headache	NB 3.1		
Hyperemia	NI 5.9.1		
Hyperlipidemia	NI 5.6.2		
Hypertension	NI 4.2	NI 4.3	NI 5.4
Hyperthyroidism (pre- or untreated)	NC 3.2		
Hypertriglyceridemia, severe	NI 4.3		
Hypoglycemia	NI 5.8.3	NI 5.8.4	
Hypothyroidism	NC 3.3	NC 3.4	
Illness, recent	NI 5.3		
Inborn errors of metabolism	NI 5.7.3		
Infection	NI 5.8.2		
Inflammatory bowel disease	NI 5.8.5	NI 5.10.1	
Irritable bowel syndrome	NI 5.4	NI 5.8.6	NC 1.4
Kidney stones	NI 5.10.1		
Lactase deficiency	NI 5.8.2		
Liver disease	NI 3.2	NI 5.2	NI 5.4
	NI 5.6.3	NI 5.8.1	NI 5.9.2
	NI 5.10.2	NB 2.3	
Malabsorption, protein and/or nutrient	NI 2.1	NI 5.7.1	NI 5.7.2
Maldigestion	NC 1.4		
Malnutrition	NI 5.2	NI 5.3	NC 3.1
Mastitis	NC 1.3		
Mental illness	NI 1.4	NI 5.8.6	NC 3.1
	NB 1.1	NB 1.2	NB 1.7
	NB 3.1	NB 3.2	
Metabolic syndrome	NI 2.2	NI 5.8.3	NI 5.8.4
Multiple sclerosis	NB 2.6		
Nephrotic syndrome	NI 3.2		
Neurological disorders	NB 2.6		
Obesity, morbid	NB 2.1		

Nutrition Assessment Matrix
Client History Data and Related Diagnostic Terminology

Parameter (not all-inclusive) Medical/Health history, cont'd	Nutrition Diagnostic Terminology		
Obesity/overweight	NI 2.2 NI 5.8.4	NI 5.6.3 NB 1.4	NI 5.8.3
Oral soft issue infection, e.g., candidiasis, leukoplakia	NC 1.2		
Osteomalacia	NI 5.9.1		
Pancreatic disease	NI 4.3	NI 5.8.1	
Paralysis	NB 2.6		
Paraplegia	NB 2.4		
Parkinson's disease	NI 1.2		
Pellegra	NI 5.9.1		
Personality disorder	NB 1.5		
Phytobezoar	NI 5.8.6		
Poisoning by drugs, medicinals or biological substances	NB 3.1		
Poisoning from food stuffs or poisonous plants	NB 3.1		
Polycystic ovary disease	NI 5.10.1		
Polyps, colon	NI 5.10.1		
Postmenopause without estrogen supplementation	NI 5.10.1		
Premature birth	NC 1.3		
Premenstrual syndrome	NI 5.10.1		
Prolapsing hemorrhoids	NI 5.8.6		
Psychiatric illness	NC 3.4		
Pulmonary failure	NI 5.3		
Rachitic rosary in children	NI 5.9.1		
Renal disease, end stage	NI 3.2	NI 5.4	NB 2.3
Rickets	NI 5.9.1		
Rheumatic conditions	NC 3.4		
Seizure disorder	NI 5.8.1		
Sepsis or severe infection	NI 5.6.1	NI 5.8.2	NI 5.8.5
Short bowel syndrome	NI 5.8.6	NI 5.9.1	NI 5.10.1
SIADH	NI 3.2		
Stroke	NB 2.6		
Tardive dyskinesia	NB 2.6		
Thrush	NC 1.3		
Trauma	NC 3.2		
Tremors	NB 2.6		
Tuberculosis	NI 2.1	NI 5.6.1	
Ulcer disease	NI 5.8.5	NI 5.8.6	
Upper respiratory infections or pneumonia	NC 1.1		
Vagotomy	NC 1.4		
Vision problems	NB 2.4	NB 3.1	
Weight loss	NB 2.6		
Wired jaw	NC 1.2		

ASSESSMENT

Edition: 2008

Nutrition Assessment Matrix
Client History Data and Related Diagnostic Terminology

Parameter (not all-inclusive)	Nutrition Diagnostic Terminology		
Mental status			
Evidence of addictive, obsessive, or compulsive tendencies	NB 2.2		
Signs and symptoms			
Abdominal cramping	NI 5.8.6		
Abdominal pain	NC 2.1	NC 1.4	
Achalasia	NC 1.1		
Acute or chronic pain	NI 1.4	NI 2.1	
Amenorrhea	NB 2.2		
Angina	NI 5.6.2		
Anorexia	NC 1.4		
Bloating	NB 3.1		
Chills	NB 3.1		
Cholesterol, serum	NI 4.1	NI 4.2	
Constipation	NC 1.4		
Contributes to the development of anemia	NI 5.5		
Cramping	NB 3.1		
Diarrhea	NI 5.5 NI 5.8.6 NC 1.4	NI 5.6.2 NC 2.1	NI 5.6.3 NB 3.1
Discomfort or pain associated with intake of foods rich in bioactive substances	NI 4.2		
Dizziness	NB 3.1		
Dysphagia	NC 3.2		
Engorgement	NC 1.3		
Enteral or parenteral nutrition intolerance	NI 2.5		
Epigastric pain	NI 5.5	NI 5.6.2	NI 5.6.3
Falls, unexplained	NI 4.3		
Feeding tube or venous access in the wrong position or removed	NI 2.3		
Fever	NB 3.1		
Flatulence, excessive	NI 5.8.6		
Gastrointestinal disturbances	NI 5.10.2		
High stool volume or frequency that causes discomfort to the individual	NI 5.8.6		
Hunger, use of alcohol or drugs that reduce hunger	NI 1.4	NI 2.1	NI 5.2
Muscle weakness	NC 3.4		
Muscle weakness, fatigue, cardiac arrhythmia, dehydration, and electrolyte imbalance	NB 1.5		
Nausea	NI 5.5 NC 1.4	NI 5.8.6	NB 3.1
Oral manifestations of systemic disease	NC 1.2		
Report of always feeling cold	NB 1.5		
Self-induced vomiting, diarrhea, bloating, constipation, flatulence	NB 1.5		

Nutrition Assessment Matrix
Client History Data and Related Diagnostic Terminology

Parameter (not all-inclusive)	Nutrition Diagnostic Terminology		
Signs and symptoms, cont'd			
Shortness of breath, dyspnea on exertion/ rest	NI 3.2	NB 2.6	
Steatorrhea	NI 5.6.2	NC 1.4	
Stool volume, low	NI 5.8.5		
Vomiting	NI 5.5 NC 1.4	NI 5.8.6	NB 3.1
Treatments			
Bowel resection	NC 1.4	NC 2.1	
Chemotherapy with oral side effects	NC 1.2		
Enteral or parenteral nutrition therapy	NI 5.7.3		
Esophagostomy or esophageal dilatation	NC 1.4		
Gastrectomy	NC 1.4		
Gastric bypass	NC 1.4	NC 2.1	
Intestinal resection	NI 2.3		
Knee surgery	NB 2.1		
Oral surgery, recent major	NC 1.2		
Ostomy, new	NB 1.4		
Radiation therapy	NC 1.2	NC 2.1	
Rigorous therapy regimen	NB 2.4		
Surgery	NI 5.3	NC 3.2	NB 2.4
Surgery requiring recumbent position	NB 2.6		
Medications and supplements			
Insulin or insulin secretagogues	NI 5.8.4		
Medications that cause somnolence and decreased cognition	NB 2.1		
Medication associated with weight loss	NC 3.2		
Medication, lipid lowering	NI 5.6.2		
Medications administered in large amounts of fluid	NI 3.2		
Medications affecting absorption or metabolism	NI 5.1		
Medications associated with increased appetite	NC 3.4		
Medications that affect appetite	NI 1.4	NC 3.1	
Medications that cause altered glucose levels	NI 5.8.2	NI 5.8.3	NI 5.8.4
Medications that cause anorexia	NI 2.1		
Medications that impact RMR	NC 3.3		
Medications that impair fluid excretion	NI 3.2		
Medications that increase energy expenditure	NI 1.2		
Medications that reduce requirements or impair metabolism of energy, protein, fat or fluid	NI 2.4		
Medications that reduce thirst	NI 3.1		

Edition: 2008

Nutrition Assessment Matrix
Client History Data and Related Diagnostic Terminology

Parameter (not all-inclusive)	Nutrition Diagnostic Terminology
Medications and supplements, cont'd	
Medications that require nutrient supplementation that cannot be accomplished with food intake	NC 2.3
Medications with known food-medication interactions	NC 2.3
Misuse of laxatives, enemas, diuretics, stimulants, and/or metabolic enhancers	NB 1.5

Updated: 2008 Edition

SNAPshot
NCP Step 2. Nutrition Diagnosis

What is the purpose of a Nutrition Diagnosis? The purpose is to identify and describe a specific nutrition problem that can be resolved or improved through treatment/nutrition intervention by a dietetic practitioner. A nutrition diagnosis (e.g., inconsistent carbohydrate intake) is different from a medical diagnosis (e.g., diabetes).

How does a dietetics practitioner determine a Nutrition Diagnosis? Dietetics practitioners use the data collected in the nutrition assessment to identify and label the patient/client's* nutrition diagnosis using standard nutrition diagnostic terminology. Each nutrition diagnosis has a reference sheet that includes its definition, possible etiology/causes and common signs or symptoms identified in the nutrition assessment step.

How are the Nutrition Diagnoses organized? In three categories.

Intake—*Too much or too little of a food or nutrient compared to actual or estimated needs*

Clinical—*Nutrition problems that relate to medical or physical conditions*

Behavioral-Environmental—*Knowledge, attitudes, beliefs, physical environment, access to food, or food safety*

How is the Nutrition Diagnosis documented? Dietetics practitioners write a PES statement to describe the problem, its root cause, and the assessment data that provide evidence for the nutrition diagnosis. The format for the PES statement is "Nutrition problem label related to _____ as evidenced by _____".

(P) Problem or Nutrition Diagnosis Label—Describes alterations in the patient/client's nutrition status.

(E) Etiology—Cause/Contributing Risk Factors (Linked to the nutrition diagnosis label by the words "related to.")

(S) Signs/Symptoms—Data used to determine that the patient/client has the nutrition diagnosis specified. (Linked to the etiology by the words "as evidenced by.")

What are the guidelines for selecting the diagnoses and writing a clear PES statement? The most important and urgent problem to be addressed is selected. When specifying the nutrition diagnosis and writing the PES statement; dietetics practitioners ask themselves a series of questions that help clarify the nutrition diagnosis. (See the critical thinking box on the next page).

Patient/client refers to individuals, groups, family members, and/or caregivers.

Edition: 2008

> **Critical thinking during this step...**
>
> Evaluate your PES statement by using the following
>
> **P** — Can the nutrition professional resolve or improve the nutrition diagnosis for this individual, group or population? When all things are equal and there is a choice between stating the PES statement using two nutrition diagnoses from different domains, consider the Intake nutrition diagnosis as the one more specific to the role of the RD.
>
> **E** — Evaluate what you have used as your etiology to determine if it is the root cause or the most specific root cause that the RD can address with a nutrition intervention. If as an RD you can not resolve the problem by addressing the etiology, can the RD intervention at least lessen the signs and symptoms?
>
> **S** — Will measuring the signs and symptoms indicate if the problem is resolved or improved? Are the signs and symptoms specific enough that you can monitor (measure/ evaluate changes) and document resolution or improvement of the nutrition diagnosis?
>
> **PES Overall** — Does the nutrition assessment data support a particular nutrition diagnosis with a typical etiology and signs and symptoms?

Are dietetics practitioners limited to the Nutrition Diagnoses terms?

Nutrition diagnosis terms and definitions were developed with extensive input and should fit most situations; however, food and dietetics practitioners can submit proposals for additions or revisions using the Procedure for Nutrition Controlled Vocabulary/Terminology Maintenance/Review available from ADA.

Detailed information about this step can be found in the International Dietetics and Nutrition Terminology (IDNT) Reference Manual: Standardized Language for the Nutrition Care Process, First Edition, American Dietetic Association.

INCREASED ENERGY EXPENDITURE (NI-1.2)

Definition
Resting metabolic rate (RMR) more than predicted requirements due to body composition, medications, endocrine, neurologic, or genetic changes. Note: RMR is the sum of metabolic processes of active cell mass related to the maintenance of normal body functions and regulatory balance during rest.

Etiology (*Cause/Contributing Risk Factors*)
Factors gathered during the nutrition assessment process that contribute to the existence or the maintenance of pathophysiological, psychosocial, situational, developmental, cultural, and/or environmental problems:
- Anabolism or growth
- Voluntary or involuntary physical activity/movement

Signs/Symptoms (*Defining Characteristics*)
A typical cluster of subjective and objective signs and symptoms gathered during the nutrition assessment process that provide evidence that a problem exists; quantify the problem and describe its severity.

Nutrition Assessment Category	Potential Indicators of this Nutrition Diagnosis (one or more must be present)
Biochemical Data, Medical Tests and Procedures	
Anthropometric Measurements	▪ Unintentional weight loss of ≥ 10% in 6 months, ≥ 5% in 1 month (adults and pediatrics) and > 2% in 1 week (pediatrics) ▪ Evidence of need for accelerated or catch-up growth or weight gain in children; absence of normal growth ▪ Increased proportional lean body mass
Physical Examination Findings	▪ Fever ▪ Measured RMR > estimated or expected RMR
Food/Nutrition History	▪ Increased physical activity, e.g., endurance athlete
Client History	▪ Conditions associated with a diagnosis or treatment, e.g., Parkinson's disease, cerebral palsy, Alzheimer's disease, cystic fibrosis, chronic obstructive pulmonary disease (COPD) ▪ Medications that increase energy expenditure

Updated: 2008 Edition

INADEQUATE ENERGY INTAKE (NI-1.4)

Definition

Energy intake that is less than energy expenditure, established reference standards, or recommendations based on physiological needs. Exception: when the goal is weight loss or during end-of-life care.

Etiology (Cause/Contributing Risk Factors)

Factors gathered during the nutrition assessment process that contribute to the existence or the maintenance of pathophysiological, psychosocial, situational, developmental, cultural, and/or environmental problems:

- Pathologic or physiological causes that result in increased energy requirements or decreased ability to consume sufficient energy, e.g., increased nutrient needs due to prolonged catabolic illness
- Lack of access to food or artificial nutrition, e.g., economic constraints, cultural, or religious practices restricting food given to elderly and/or children
- Food- and nutrition-related knowledge deficit
- Psychological causes, e.g., depression or disordered eating

Signs/Symptoms (Defining Characteristics)

A typical cluster of subjective and objective signs and symptoms gathered during the nutrition assessment process that provide evidence that a problem exists; quantify the problem and describe its severity.

Nutrition Assessment Category	Potential Indicators of this Nutrition Diagnosis (one or more must be present)
Biochemical Data, Medical Tests and Procedures	
Anthropometric Measurements	
Physical Examination Findings	▪ Failure to gain or maintain appropriate weight ▪ Poor dentition

INADEQUATE ENERGY INTAKE (NI-1.4)

Food/Nutrition History	Reports or observations of: ▪ Insufficient energy intake from diet compared to needs based on estimated or measured resting metabolic rate ▪ Restriction or omission of energy-dense foods from diet ▪ Food avoidance and/or lack of interest in food ▪ Inability to independently consume foods/fluids (diminished joint mobility of wrist, hand, or digits) ▪ Parenteral or enteral nutrition insufficient to meet needs based on estimated or measured resting metabolic rate
Client History	▪ Excessive consumption of alcohol or other drugs that reduce hunger ▪ Conditions associated with diagnosis or treatment, e.g., mental illness, eating disorders, dementia, alcoholism, substance abuse, and acute or chronic pain management ▪ Medications that affect appetite

Updated: 2008 Edition

INTAKE

EXCESSIVE ENERGY INTAKE (NI-1.5)

Definition

Energy intake (e.g., oral, EN/PN, IV, medications) that exceeds energy expenditure, established reference standards, or recommendations based on physiological needs. Exception: when weight gain is desired.

Etiology (*Cause/Contributing Risk Factors*)

Factors gathered during the nutrition assessment process that contribute to the existence or the maintenance of pathophysiological, psychosocial, situational, developmental, cultural, and/or environmental problems:

- Harmful beliefs/attitudes about food, nutrition, and nutrition-related topics
- Food- and nutrition-related knowledge deficit
- Lack of access to healthful food choices, e.g., healthful food choices not provided as an option by caregiver or parent, homeless
- Lack of value for behavior change, competing values
- Medications that increase appetite, e.g., steroids, antidepressants
- Overfeeding of parenteral/enteral nutrition (PN/EN)
- Calories unaccounted for from IV infusion and/or medications
- Unwilling or uninterested in reducing energy intake
- Failure to adjust for lifestyle changes and decreased metabolism (e.g., aging)
- Resolution of prior hypermetabolism without reduction in intake

Signs/Symptoms (*Defining Characteristics*)

A typical cluster of subjective and objective signs and symptoms gathered during the nutrition assessment process that provide evidence that a problem exists; quantify the problem and describe its severity.

Nutrition Assessment Category	Potential Indicators of this Nutrition Diagnosis (one or more must be present)
Biochemical Data, Medical Tests and Procedures	▪ Abnormal liver function tests after prolonged exposure (3-6 weeks) ▪ Respiratory quotient >1.0
Anthropometric Measurements	▪ Body fat percentage > 25% for men and > 32% for women ▪ BMI > 25 (adults), BMI > 95th percentile (pediatrics) ▪ Weight gain
Physical Exam Findings	▪ Increased body adiposity ▪ Increased respiratory rate
Food/Nutrition History	Reports or observations of: ▪ Intake of high caloric density or large portions of foods/beverages ▪ EN/PN more than estimated or measured (e.g., indirect calorimetry) energy expenditure
Client History	

Updated: 2008 Edition

INADEQUATE ORAL FOOD/BEVERAGE INTAKE (NI-2.1)

Definition
Oral food/beverage intake that is less than established reference standards or recommendations based on physiological needs. Exception: when the goal is weight loss or during end-of-life care.

Etiology (*Cause/Contributing Risk Factors*)
Factors gathered during the nutrition assessment process that contribute to the existence or the maintenance of pathophysiological, psychosocial, situational, developmental, cultural, and/or environmental problems:

- Physiological causes, e.g., increased nutrient needs due to prolonged catabolic illness
- Lack of access to food, e.g., economic constraints, cultural or religious practices, restricting food given to elderly and/or children
- Food- and nutrition-related knowledge deficit concerning sufficient oral food/beverage intake
- Psychological causes, e.g., depression or disordered eating

Signs/Symptoms (*Defining Characteristics*)
A typical cluster of subjective and objective signs and symptoms gathered during the nutrition assessment process that provide evidence that a problem exists; quantify the problem and describe its severity.

Nutrition Assessment Category	Potential Indicators of this Nutrition Diagnosis (one or more must be present)
Biochemical Data, Medical Tests and Procedures	
Anthropometric Measurements	▪ Weight loss, insufficient growth velocity
Physical Examination Findings	▪ Dry skin, mucous membranes, poor skin turgor
Food/Nutrition History	Reports or observations of: ▪ Insufficient intake of energy or high-quality protein from diet when compared to requirements ▪ Economic constraints that limit food availability ▪ Anorexia, nausea, or vomiting ▪ Change in appetite or taste
Client History	▪ Conditions associated with a diagnosis or treatment of catabolic illness such as AIDS, tuberculosis, anorexia nervosa, sepsis or infection from recent surgery, depression, acute or chronic pain ▪ Protein and/or nutrient malabsorption ▪ Excessive consumption of alcohol or other drugs that reduce hunger ▪ Medications that cause anorexia

INTAKE

EXCESSIVE ORAL FOOD/BEVERAGE INTAKE (NI-2.2)

Definition

Oral food/beverage intake that exceeds estimated energy needs, established reference standards, or recommendations based on physiological needs. Exception: when weight gain is desired.

Etiology (*Cause/Contributing Risk Factors*)

Factors gathered during the nutrition assessment process that contribute to the existence or the maintenance of pathophysiological, psychosocial, situational, developmental, cultural, and/or environmental problems:

- Harmful beliefs/attitudes about food, nutrition, and nutrition-related topics
- Food- and nutrition-related knowledge deficit
- Lack of access to healthful food choices, e.g., healthful food choices not provided as an option by caregiver or parent, homeless
- Lack of value for behavior change, competing values
- Inability to limit or refuse offered foods
- Lack of food planning, purchasing, and preparation skills
- Loss of appetite awareness
- Medications that increase appetite, e.g., steroids, antidepressants
- Mental illness, depression
- Unwilling or uninterested in reducing intake

Signs/Symptoms (*Defining Characteristics*)

A typical cluster of subjective and objective signs and symptoms gathered during the nutrition assessment process that provide evidence that a problem exists; quantify the problem and describe its severity.

Nutrition Assessment Category	Potential Indicators of this Nutrition Diagnosis (one or more must be present)
Biochemical Data, Medical Tests and Procedures	
Anthropometric Measurements	▪ Weight gain not attributed to fluid retention or normal growth
Physical Exam Findings	
Food/Nutrition History	Reports or observations of: ▪ Intake of high caloric-density foods/beverages (juice, soda, or alcohol) at meals and/or snacks ▪ Intake of large portions of foods/beverages, food groups, or specific food items ▪ Intake that exceeds estimated or measured energy needs ▪ Highly variable daily energy intake ▪ Binge eating patterns ▪ Frequent, excessive fast food or restaurant intake
Client History	▪ Conditions associated with a diagnosis or treatment, e.g., obesity, overweight, or metabolic syndrome, depression, anxiety disorder

INADEQUATE INTAKE FROM ENTERAL/PARENTERAL (EN/PN) NUTRITION (NI-2.3)

Definition

Enteral or parenteral infusion that provides fewer calories or nutrients compared to established reference standards or recommendations based on physiological needs. Exception: when recommendation is for weight loss or during end-of-life care.

Etiology (*Cause/Contributing Risk Factors*)

Factors gathered during the nutrition assessment process that contribute to the existence or the maintenance of pathophysiological, psychosocial, situational, developmental, cultural, and/or environmental problems:

- Altered absorption or metabolism of nutrients, e.g., medications
- Food- and nutrition-related knowledge deficit (patient/client, caregiver, supplier)—incorrect formula/formulation given, e.g., wrong enteral feeding, missing component of PN
- Lack of, compromised, or incorrect access for delivering EN/PN
- Increased biological demand of nutrients, e.g., accelerated growth, wound healing, chronic infection, multiple fractures
- Intolerance of EN/PN
- Infusion volume not reached or schedule for infusion interrupted

Signs/Symptoms (*Defining Characteristics*)

A typical cluster of subjective and objective signs and symptoms gathered during the nutrition assessment process that provide evidence that a problem exists; quantify the problem and describe its severity.

Nutrition Assessment Category	Potential Indicators of this Nutrition Diagnosis (one or more must be present)
Biochemical Data, Medical Tests and Procedures	▪ Metabolic cart/indirect calorimetry measurement, e.g., respiratory quotient < 0.7 ▪ Vitamin/mineral abnormalities: • Calcium < 9.2 mg/dL (2.3 mmol/L) • Vitamin K—abnormal international normalized ratio (INR) • Copper < 70 µg/dL (11 µmol/L) • Zinc < 78 µg/dL (12 µmol/L) • Iron < 50 µg/dL(nmol/L); iron-binding capacity < 250 µg/dL (44.8 µmol/L)

Edition: 2008

INADEQUATE INTAKE FROM ENTERAL/PARENTERAL (EN/PN) NUTRITION CONT'D (NI-2.3)

Anthropometric Measurements	▪ Growth failure, based on National Center for Health Statistics (NCHS) growth standards and fetal growth failure ▪ Insufficient maternal weight gain ▪ Lack of planned weight gain ▪ Unintentional weight loss of ≥ 5% in 1 month or ≥ 10% in 6 months (not attributed to fluid) in adults ▪ Any weight loss in infants or children ▪ Underweight (BMI < 18.5)
Physical Exam Findings	▪ Clinical evidence of vitamin/mineral deficiency (e.g., hair loss, bleeding gums, pale nail beds, neurologic changes) ▪ Evidence of dehydration, e.g., dry mucous membranes, poor skin turgor ▪ Loss of skin integrity, delayed wound healing, or pressure ulcers ▪ Loss of muscle mass and/or subcutaneous fat ▪ Nausea, vomiting, diarrhea
Food/Nutrition History	Reports or observations of: ▪ Inadequate EN/PN volume compared to estimated or measured (indirect calorimetry) requirements
Client History	▪ Conditions associated with a diagnosis or treatment, e.g., intestinal resection, Crohn's disease, HIV/AIDS, burns, pre-term birth, malnutrition ▪ Feeding tube or venous access in wrong position or removed ▪ Altered capacity for desired levels of physical activity or exercise, easy fatigue with increased activity

Updated: 2008 Edition

EXCESSIVE INTAKE FROM ENTERAL OR PARENTERAL NUTRITION (NI-2.4)

Definition

Enteral or parenteral infusion that provides more calories or nutrients compared to established reference standards or recommendations based on physiological needs.

Etiology (*Cause/Contributing Risk Factors*)

Factors gathered during the nutrition assessment process that contribute to the existence or the maintenance of pathophysiological, psychosocial, situational, developmental, cultural, and/or environmental problems:

- Physiological causes, e.g., decreased needs related to low activity levels with critical illness or organ failure
- Food- and nutrition-related knowledge deficit on the part of the caregiver, patient/client, or clinician

Signs/Symptoms (*Defining Characteristics*)

A typical cluster of subjective and objective signs and symptoms gathered during the nutrition assessment process that provide evidence that a problem exists; quantify the problem and describe its severity.

Nutrition Assessment Category	Potential Indicators of this Nutrition Diagnosis (one or more must be present)
Biochemical Data, Medical Tests and Procedures	▪ Elevated BUN:creatinine ratio (protein) ▪ Hyperglycemia (carbohydrate) ▪ Hypercapnia ▪ Elevated liver enzymes
Anthropometric Measurements	▪ Weight gain in excess of lean tissue accretion
Physical Examination Findings	▪ Edema with excess fluid administration
Food/Nutrition History	Reports or observations of: ▪ Documented intake from enteral or parenteral nutrients that is consistently more than recommended intake for carbohydrate, protein, and fat (e.g., 36 kcal/kg for well, active adults, 25 kcal/kg or as measured by indirect calorimetry for critically ill adults, 0.8 g/kg protein for well adults, 1.5 g/kg protein for critically ill adults, 4 mg/kg/minute of dextrose for critically ill adults, 1.2 g/kg lipid for adults, or 3 g/kg for children)*
Client History	▪ Use of drugs that reduce requirements or impair metabolism of energy, protein, fat, or fluid. ▪ Unrealistic expectations of weight gain or ideal weight

* When entering weight (i.e., gram) information into the medical record, use institution or Joint Commission approved abbreviation list.

Edition: 2008

INAPPROPRIATE INFUSION OF ENTERAL OR PARENTERAL NUTRITION (NI-2.5)

Use with caution–only after discussion with other health team members

Definition

Enteral or parenteral infusion that provides either fewer or more calories and/or nutrients or is of the wrong composition or type, parenteral or enteral nutrition that is not warranted because the patient/client is able to tolerate an enteral intake, or is unsafe because of the potential for sepsis or other complications.

Etiology *(Cause/Contributing Risk Factors)*

Factors gathered during the nutrition assessment process that contribute to the existence or the maintenance of pathophysiological, psychosocial, situational, developmental, cultural, and/or environmental problems:

- Physiological causes, e.g., improvement in patient/client status, allowing return to total or partial oral diet; changes in the course of disease resulting in changes in nutrient requirements
- Product or knowledge deficit on the part of the caregiver or clinician
- End-of-life care if patient/client or family do not desire nutrition support

Signs/Symptoms *(Defining Characteristics)*

A typical cluster of subjective and objective signs and symptoms gathered during the nutrition assessment process that provide evidence that a problem exists; quantify the problem and describe its severity.

Nutrition Assessment Category	Potential Indicators of this Nutrition Diagnosis (one or more must be present)
Biochemical Data, Medical Tests and Procedures	▪ Abnormal liver function tests in patient/client on long-term (more than 3-6 weeks) feeding ▪ Abnormal levels of markers specific for various nutrients, e.g., hyperphosphatemia in patient/client receiving feedings with a high phosphorus content, hypokalemia in patient/client receiving feedings with low potassium content
Anthropometric Measurements	▪ Weight gain in excess of lean tissue accretion ▪ Weight loss
Physical Examination Findings	▪ Edema with excess fluid administration ▪ Loss of subcutaneous fat and muscle stores

INTAKE

INAPPROPRIATE INFUSION OF ENTERAL OR PARENTERAL NUTRITION (NI-2.5)

Food/Nutrition History	Reports or observations of: • Documented intake from enteral or parenteral nutrients that is consistently more or less than recommended intake for carbohydrate, protein, and/or fat—especially related to patient/client's ability to consume an oral diet that meets needs at this point in time • Documented intake of other nutrients that is consistently more or less than recommended • Nausea, vomiting, diarrhea, high gastric residual volume
Client History	• History of enteral or parenteral nutrition intolerance • Complications such as fatty liver in the absence of other causes

Edition: 2008

INADEQUATE FLUID INTAKE (NI-3.1)

Definition
Lower intake of fluid-containing foods or substances compared to established reference standards or recommendations based on physiological needs.

Etiology (*Cause/Contributing Risk Factors*)
Factors gathered during the nutrition assessment process that contribute to the existence or the maintenance of pathophysiological, psychosocial, situational, developmental, cultural, and/or environmental problems:

- Physiological causes, e.g., increased fluid needs due to climate/ temperature change; increased exercise or conditions leading to increased fluid losses; fever causing increased insensible losses, decreased thirst sensation, use of drugs that reduce thirst
- Lack of access to fluid, e.g., economic constraints, cultural or religious practices, unable to access fluid independently such as elderly or children
- Food- and nutrition-related knowledge deficit
- Psychological causes, e.g., depression or disordered eating; dementia resulting in decreased recognition of thirst

Signs/Symptoms (*Defining Characteristics*)
A typical cluster of subjective and objective signs and symptoms gathered during the nutrition assessment process that provide evidence that a problem exists; quantify the problem and describe its severity.

Nutrition Assessment Category	Potential Indicators of this Nutrition Diagnosis (one or more must be present)
Biochemical Data, Medical Tests and Procedures	▪ Plasma or serum osmolality greater than 290 mOsm/kg ▪ ↑ BUN, ↑ Na
Anthropometric Measurements	▪ Acute weight loss
Physical Examination Findings	▪ Dry skin and mucous membranes, poor skin turgor ▪ Urine output <30 mL/hr
Food/Nutrition History	Reports or observations of: ▪ Insufficient intake of fluid compared to requirements (e.g., per body surface area for pediatrics) ▪ Thirst ▪ Difficulty swallowing
Client History	▪ Conditions associated with a diagnosis or treatment, e.g., Alzheimer's disease or other dementia resulting in decreased recognition of thirst, diarrhea ▪ Use of drugs that reduce thirst

Updated: 2008 Edition

EXCESSIVE FLUID INTAKE (NI-3.2)

Definition

Higher intake of fluid compared to established reference standards or recommendations based on physiological needs.

Etiology (*Cause/Contributing Risk Factors*)

Factors gathered during the nutrition assessment process that contribute to the existence or the maintenance of pathophysiological, psychosocial, situational, developmental, cultural, and/or environmental problems:

- Physiological causes, e.g., decreased fluid losses due to kidney, liver or cardiac failure; diminished water and sodium losses due to changes in exercise or climate, syndrome of inappropriate antidiuretic hormone (SIADH)
- Food- and nutrition-related knowledge deficit
- Psychological causes, e.g., depression or disordered eating

Signs/Symptoms (*Defining Characteristics*)

A typical cluster of subjective and objective signs and symptoms gathered during the nutrition assessment process that provide evidence that a problem exists; quantify the problem and describe its severity.

Nutrition Assessment Category	Potential Indicators of this Nutrition Diagnosis (one or more must be present)
Biochemical Data, Medical Tests and Procedures	■ Lowered plasma osmolarity (270-280 mOsm/kg), only if positive fluid balance is in excess of positive sodium balance ■ Decreased serum sodium in SIADH
Anthropometric Measurements	■ Weight gain
Physical Examination Findings	■ Edema in the skin of the legs, sacral area, or diffusely; weeping of fluids from lower legs ■ Ascites ■ Pulmonary edema as evidenced by shortness of breath; orthopnea; crackles or rales
Food/Nutrition History	Reports or observations of: ■ Excessive intake of fluid compared to requirements (e.g., per body surface area for pediatrics) ■ Excessive salt intake
Client History	■ Conditions associated with a diagnosis or treatment, e.g., end-stage renal disease, nephrotic syndrome, heart failure, or liver disease ■ Nausea, vomiting, anorexia, headache, muscle spasms, convulsions, coma (SIADH) ■ Shortness of breath or dyspnea with exertion or at rest ■ Providing medications in large amounts of fluid ■ Use of drugs that impair fluid excretion

Updated: 2008 Edition

INADEQUATE BIOACTIVE SUBSTANCE INTAKE (NI-4.1)

Definition
Lower intake of bioactive substances or foods containing bioactive substances compared to established reference standards or recommendations based on physiological needs.

*Bioactive substances are the physiologically active components of foods

Etiology (Cause/Contributing Risk Factors)
Factors gathered during the nutrition assessment process that contribute to the existence or the maintenance of pathophysiological, psychosocial, situational, developmental, cultural, and/or environmental problems:

- Food- and nutrition-related knowledge deficit
- Limited access to a food that contains the substance
- Altered GI function, e.g., pain or discomfort

Signs/Symptoms (Defining Characteristics)
A typical cluster of subjective and objective signs and symptoms gathered during the nutrition assessment process that provide evidence that a problem exists; quantify the problem and describe its severity.

Nutrition Assessment Category	Potential Indicators of this Nutrition Diagnosis (one or more must be present)
Biochemical Data, Medical Tests and Procedures	
Anthropometric Measurements	
Physical Exam Findings	
Food/Nutrition History	Reports or observations of: • Low intake of plant foods containing: ▪ Soluble fiber, e.g., psyllium (↓ total and LDL cholesterol) ▪ Soy protein (↓ total and LDL cholesterol) ▪ β-glucan, e.g., whole oat products (↓ total and LDL cholesterol) ▪ Plant sterol and stanol esters, e.g., fortified margarines (↓ total and LDL cholesterol)
Client History	▪ Conditions associated with a diagnosis or treatment, e.g., cardiovascular disease, elevated cholesterol

Updated: 2008 Edition

EXCESSIVE BIOACTIVE SUBSTANCE INTAKE (NI-4.2)

Definition

Higher intake of bioactive substances other than traditional nutrients, such as functional foods, bioactive food components, dietary supplements, food concentrates compared to established reference standards or recommendations based on physiological needs.

*Bioactive substances are the physiologically active components of foods

Etiology *(Cause/Contributing Risk Factors)*

Factors gathered during the nutrition assessment process that contribute to the existence or the maintenance of pathophysiological, psychosocial, situational, developmental, cultural, and/or environmental problems:

- Food- and nutrition-related knowledge deficit
- Contamination, misname, mislabel, misuse, recent brand change, recent dose increase, recent formulation change of substance consumed
- Frequent intake of foods containing bioactive substances
- Altered GI function, e.g., pain or discomfort

Signs/Symptoms *(Defining Characteristics)*

A typical cluster of subjective and objective signs and symptoms gathered during the nutrition assessment process that provide evidence that a problem exists; quantify the problem and describe its severity.

Nutrition Assessment Category	Potential Indicators of this Nutrition Diagnosis (one or more must be present)
Biochemical Data, Medical Tests and Procedures	▪ Lab values indicating excessive intake of the specific substance, such as rapid decrease in cholesterol from intake of stanol or sterol esters and a statin drug and related dietary changes or medications ▪ Increased hepatic enzyme reflecting hepatocellular damage
Anthropometric Measurements	▪ Weight loss as a result of malabsorption or maldigestion
Physical Exam Findings	▪ Constipation or diarrhea related to excessive intake ▪ Neurologic changes, e.g., anxiety, mental status changes ▪ Cardiovascular changes, e.g., heart rate, EKG changes, blood pressure

Edition: 2008

EXCESSIVE BIOACTIVE SUBSTANCE INTAKE CONT'D (NI-4.2)

Food/Nutrition History	Reports or observations of:
	▪ High intake of plant foods containing:
	  • Soy protein (↓ total and LDL cholesterol)
	  • β-glucan, e.g., whole oat products (↓ total and LDL cholesterol)
	  • Plant sterol and stanol esters, e.g., fortified margarines (↓ total and LDL cholesterol) or other foods based on dietary substance, concentrate, metabolite, constituent, extract, or combination
	  • Substances that interfere with digestion or absorption of foodstuffs
	▪ Ready access to available foods/products with bioactive substance, e.g., as from dietary supplement vendors
	▪ Attempts to use supplements or bioactive substances for weight loss, to treat constipation, or to prevent or cure chronic or acute disease

Client History	▪ Conditions associated with a diagnosis or treatment, e.g., cardiovascular disease, elevated cholesterol, hypertension ▪ Discomfort or pain associated with intake of foods rich in bioactive substances, e.g., soluble fiber, β-glucan, soy protein

Updated: 2008 Edition

EXCESSIVE ALCOHOL INTAKE (NI-4.3)

Definition
Intake more than the suggested limits for alcohol.

Etiology *(Cause/Contributing Risk Factors)*
Factors gathered during the nutrition assessment process that contribute to the existence or the maintenance of pathophysiological, psychosocial, situational, developmental, cultural, and/or environmental problems:

- Harmful beliefs/attitudes about food, nutrition, and nutrition-related topics
- Food- and nutrition-related knowledge deficit
- Lack of value for behavior change, competing values
- Alcohol addiction

Signs/Symptoms *(Defining Characteristics)*
A typical cluster of subjective and objective signs and symptoms gathered during the nutrition assessment process that provide evidence that a problem exists; quantify the problem and describe its severity.

Nutrition Assessment Category	Potential Indicators of this Nutrition Diagnosis (one or more must be present)
Biochemical Data, Medical Tests and Procedures	▪ Elevated aspartate aminotransferase (AST), gamma-glutamyl transferase (GGT), carbohydrate-deficient transferrin, mean corpuscular volume, blood alcohol levels
Anthropometric Measurements	
Physical Exam Findings	
Food/Nutrition History	Reports or observations of: ▪ Intake of > 2 drinks*/day (men) ▪ Intake of > 1 drink*/day (women) ▪ Binge drinking ▪ Consumption of any alcohol when contraindicated *1 drink = 5 oz wine, 12 oz beer, 1 oz distilled alcohol
Client History	▪ Conditions associated with a diagnosis or treatment, e.g., severe hypertriglyceridemia, elevated blood pressure, depression, liver disease, pancreatitis ▪ New medical diagnosis or change in existing diagnosis or condition ▪ History of excessive alcohol intake ▪ Giving birth to an infant with fetal alcohol syndrome ▪ Drinking during pregnancy despite knowledge of risk

INTAKE

Updated: 2008 Edition

INCREASED NUTRIENT NEEDS (SPECIFY) (NI-5.1)

Definition
Increased need for a specific nutrient compared to established reference standards or recommendations based on physiological needs.

Etiology (*Cause/Contributing Risk Factors*)
Factors gathered during the nutrition assessment process that contribute to the existence or the maintenance of pathophysiological, psychosocial, situational, developmental, cultural, and/or environmental problems:

- Altered absorption or metabolism of nutrient, e.g., from medications
- Compromise of organs related to GI function, e.g., pancreas, liver
- Decreased functional length of intestine, e.g., short-bowel syndrome
- Decreased or compromised function of intestine, e.g., celiac disease, Crohn's disease
- Food- and nutrition-related knowledge deficit
- Increased demand for nutrient, e.g., accelerated growth, wound healing, chronic infection

Signs/Symptoms (*Defining Characteristics*)
A typical cluster of subjective and objective signs and symptoms gathered during the nutrition assessment process that provide evidence that a problem exists; quantify the problem and describe its severity.

Nutrition Assessment Category	Potential Indicators of this Nutrition Diagnosis (one or more must be present)
Biochemical Data, Medical Tests and Procedures	• Decreased total cholesterol < 160 mg/dL, albumin, prealbumin, C-reactive protein, indicating increased stress and increased metabolic needs • Electrolyte/mineral (e.g., potassium, magnesium, phosphorus) abnormalities • Urinary or fecal losses of specific or related nutrient (e.g., fecal fat, d-xylose test) • Vitamin and/or mineral deficiency
Anthropometric Measurements	• Growth failure, based on National Center for Health Statistics (NCHS) growth standards and fetal growth failure • Unintentional weight loss of ≥5% in 1 month or ≥10% in 6 months • Loss of muscle mass, subcutaneous fat • Underweight (BMI < 18.5)

INCREASED NUTRIENT NEEDS (SPECIFY) (NI-5.1)

Physical Examination Findings	▪ Clinical evidence of vitamin/mineral deficiency (e.g., hair loss, bleeding gums, pale nail beds) ▪ Loss of skin integrity, delayed wound healing, or pressure ulcers
Food/Nutrition History	Reports or observations of: ▪ Inadequate intake of foods/supplement containing needed nutrient as compared to estimated requirements ▪ Intake of foods that do not contain sufficient quantities of available nutrient (e.g., overprocessed, overcooked, or stored improperly) ▪ Food- and nutrition-related knowledge deficit (e.g., lack of information, incorrect information or noncompliance with intake of needed nutrient)
Client History	▪ Conditions associated with a diagnosis or treatment, e.g., intestinal resection, Crohn's disease, HIV/AIDS, burns, pre-term birth, malnutrition ▪ Medications affecting absorption or metabolism of needed nutrient

INTAKE

Updated: 2008 Edition

EVIDENT PROTEIN–ENERGY MALNUTRITION (NI-5.2)

Definition

Inadequate intake of protein and/or energy over prolonged periods of time resulting in loss of fat stores and/or muscle wasting.

Etiology (*Cause/Contributing Risk Factors*)

Factors gathered during the nutrition assessment process that contribute to the existence or the maintenance of pathophysiological, psychosocial, situational, developmental, cultural, and/or environmental problems:

- Physiological causes, e.g., altered nutrient needs due to prolonged catabolic illness, malabsorption
- Lack of access to food, e.g., economic constraints, cultural or religious practices, restricting food given to elderly and/or children
- Food- and nutrition-related knowledge deficit, e.g., avoidance of high-quality protein foods
- Psychological causes, e.g., depression or eating disorders

Signs/Symptoms (*Defining Characteristics*)

A typical cluster of subjective and objective signs and symptoms gathered during the nutrition assessment process that provide evidence that a problem exists; quantify the problem and describe its severity.

Nutrition Assessment Category	Potential Indicators of this Nutrition Diagnosis (one or more must be present)
Biochemical Data, Medical Tests and Procedures	▪ Normal serum albumin level (uncomplicated malnutrition) ▪ Albumin < 3.4 mg/dL (disease/trauma related malnutrition)
Anthropometric Measurements	▪ BMI < 18.5 indicates underweight ▪ Failure to thrive, e.g., failure to attain desirable growth rates ▪ Inadequate maternal weight gain ▪ Weight loss of > 10% in 6 months ▪ Underweight with muscle wasting ▪ Normal or slightly underweight, stunted growth in children

EVIDENT PROTEIN–ENERGY MALNUTRITION (NI-5.2)

Physical Exam Findings	▪ Uncomplicated malnutrition: Thin, wasted appearance; severe muscle wasting; minimal body fat; sparse, thin, dry, easily pluckable hair; dry, thin skin; obvious bony prominences, occipital wasting; lowered body temperature, blood pressure, heart rate; changes in hair or nails consistent with insufficient protein intake ▪ Disease/trauma related malnutrition: Thin to normal appearance, with peripheral edema, ascites, or anasarca; edema of the lower extremities; some muscle wasting with retention of some body fat; dyspigmentation of hair (flag sign) and skin ▪ Delayed wound healing
Food/Nutrition History	Reports or observations of: ▪ Insufficient energy intake from diet compared to estimated or measured RMR ▪ Insufficient intake of high-quality protein when compared to requirements ▪ Food avoidance and/or lack of interest in food
Client History	▪ Chronic or acute disease or trauma, geographic location and socioeconomic status associated with altered nutrient intake of indigenous phenomenon ▪ Severe protein and/or nutrient malabsorption (e.g., extensive bowel resection) ▪ Excessive consumption of alcohol or other drugs that reduce hunger ▪ Enlarged fatty liver

INTAKE

Edition: 2008

INADEQUATE PROTEIN–ENERGY INTAKE (NI-5.3)

Definition

Inadequate intake of protein and/or energy compared to established reference standards or recommendations based on physiological needs of short or recent duration.

Etiology (*Cause/Contributing Risk Factors*)

Factors gathered during the nutrition assessment process that contribute to the existence or the maintenance of pathophysiological, psychosocial, situational, developmental, cultural, and/or environmental problems:

- Short-term physiological causes, e.g., increased nutrient needs due to catabolic illness, malabsorption
- Recent lack of access to food, e.g., economic constraints, cultural or religious practices, restricting food given or food selected
- Food- and nutrition-related knowledge deficit, e.g., avoidance of all fats for new dieting pattern
- Recent onset of psychological causes, e.g., depression or eating disorders

Signs/Symptoms (*Defining Characteristics*)

A typical cluster of subjective and objective signs and symptoms gathered during the nutrition assessment process that provide evidence that a problem exists; quantify the problem and describe its severity.

Nutrition Assessment Category	Potential Indicators of this Nutrition Diagnosis (one or more must be present)
Biochemical Data, Medical Tests and Procedures	▪ Normal albumin (in the setting of normal liver function despite decrease protein-energy intake)
Anthropometric Measurements	▪ Inadequate maternal weight gain (mild but not severe) ▪ Weight loss of 5%-7% during past 3 months in adults, any weight loss in children ▪ Normal or slightly underweight ▪ Growth failure in children
Physical Exam Findings	▪ Slow wound healing in pressure ulcer or surgical patient/client

INADEQUATE PROTEIN–ENERGY INTAKE (NI-5.3)

Food/Nutrition History	Reports or observations of: • Insufficient energy intake from diet compared to estimated or measured RMR or recommended levels • Restriction or omission of food groups such as dairy or meat group foods (protein); bread or milk group foods (energy) • Recent food avoidance and/or lack of interest in food • Lack of ability to prepare meals
Client History	• Conditions associated with a diagnosis or treatment of mild protein-energy malnutrition, recent illness, e.g., pulmonary or cardiac failure, flu, infection, surgery • Nutrient malabsorption (e.g., bariatric surgery, diarrhea, steatorrhea) • Excessive consumption of alcohol or other drugs that reduce hunger • Patient/client reports of hunger in the face of inadequate access to food supply • Patient/client reports lack of ability to prepare meals • Patient/client reports lack of funds for purchase of appropriate foods

INTAKE

DECREASED NUTRIENT NEEDS (SPECIFY) (NI-5.4)

Definition
Decreased need for a specific nutrient compared to established reference standards or recommendations based on physiological needs.

Etiology (*Cause/Contributing Risk Factors*)
Factors gathered during the nutrition assessment process that contribute to the existence or the maintenance of pathophysiological, psychosocial, situational, developmental, cultural, and/or environmental problems:

- Renal dysfunction
- Liver dysfunction
- Altered cholesterol metabolism/regulation
- Heart failure
- Food intolerances, e.g., irritable bowel syndrome

Signs/Symptoms (*Defining Characteristics*)
A typical cluster of subjective and objective signs and symptoms gathered during the nutrition assessment process that provide evidence that a problem exists; quantify the problem and describe its severity.

Nutrition Assessment Category	Potential Indicators of this Nutrition Diagnosis (one or more must be present)
Biochemical Data, Medical Tests and Procedures	▪ Total cholesterol > 200 mg/dL (5.2 mmol/L), LDL cholesterol > 100 mg/dL (2.59 mmol/L), HDL cholesterol < 40 mg/dL (1.036 mmol/L), triglycerides > 150 mg/dL (1.695 mmol/L) ▪ Phosphorus > 5.5 mg/dL (1.78 mmol/L) ▪ Glomerular filtration rate (GFR) < 90 mL/min/1.73 m2 ▪ Elevated BUN, creatinine, potassium ▪ Liver function tests indicating severe liver disease
Anthropometric Measurements	▪ Interdialytic weight gain greater than expected
Physical Exam Findings	▪ Edema/fluid retention
Food/Nutrition History	Reports or observations of: ▪ Intake higher than recommended for fat, phosphorus, sodium, protein, fiber
Client History	▪ Conditions associated with a diagnosis or treatment that require a specific type and/or amount of nutrient, e.g., cardiovascular disease (fat), early renal disease (protein, phos), ESRD (phos, sodium, potassium, fluid), advanced liver disease (protein), heart failure (sodium, fluid), irritable bowel disease/Crohn's flare up (fiber) ▪ Diagnosis of hypertension, confusion related to liver disease

IMBALANCE OF NUTRIENTS (NI-5.5)

Definition

An undesirable combination of ingested nutrients, such that the amount of one nutrient ingested interferes with or alters absorption and/or utilization of another nutrient.

Etiology (*Cause/Contributing Risk Factors*)

Factors gathered during the nutrition assessment process that contribute to the existence or the maintenance of pathophysiological, psychosocial, situational, developmental, cultural, and/or environmental problems:

- Consumption of high-dose nutrient supplements
- Food- and nutrition-related knowledge deficit
- Harmful beliefs/attitudes about food, nutrition, and nutrition-related information
- Food faddism
- Insufficient electrolyte replacement when initiating feeding (PN/EN, including oral)

Signs/Symptoms (*Defining Characteristics*)

A typical cluster of subjective and objective signs and symptoms gathered during the nutrition assessment process that provide evidence that a problem exists; quantify the problem and describe its severity.

Nutrition Assessment Category	Potential Indicators of this Nutrition Diagnosis (one or more must be present)
Biochemical Data, Medical Tests and Procedures	▪ Severe hypophosphatemia ($\uparrow$ carbohydrate) ▪ Severe hypokalemia ($\uparrow$ protein) ▪ Severe hypomagnesemia ($\uparrow$ carbohydrate) ▪ Refeeding syndrome
Anthropometric Data	
Physical Exam Findings	
Food/Nutrition History	Reports or observations of: ▪ High intake of iron supplements ($\downarrow$ zinc absorption) ▪ High intake of zinc supplements ($\downarrow$ copper status) ▪ High intake of manganese ($\downarrow$ iron status)
Client History	▪ Diarrhea or constipation (iron supplements) ▪ Epigastric pain, nausea, vomiting, diarrhea (zinc supplements) ▪ Contributes to the development of anemia (manganese supplements)

Updated: 2008 Edition

INADEQUATE FAT INTAKE (NI-5.6.1)

Definition

Lower fat intake compared to established reference standards or recommendations based on physiological needs. Exception: when the goal is weight loss or during end-of-life care.

Etiology (*Cause/Contributing Risk Factors*)

Factors gathered during the nutrition assessment process that contribute to the existence or the maintenance of pathophysiological, psychosocial, situational, developmental, cultural, and/or environmental problems:

- Inappropriate food choices, e.g., economic constraints, cultural or religious practices, restricting food given to elderly and/or children, specific food choices
- Food- and nutrition-related knowledge deficit, e.g., prolonged adherence to a very–low-fat diet
- Psychological causes, e.g., depression or disordered eating

Signs/Symptoms (*Defining Characteristics*)

A typical cluster of subjective and objective signs and symptoms gathered during the nutrition assessment process that provide evidence that a problem exists; quantify the problem and describe its severity.

Nutrition Assessment Category	Potential Indicators of this Nutrition Diagnosis (one or more must be present)
Biochemical Data, Medical Tests and Procedures	▪ Triene: tetraene ratio > 0.2
Anthropometric Measurements	▪ Impaired growth ▪ Weight loss if insufficient calories consumed
Physical Examination Findings	▪ Scaly skin and dermatitis consistent with essential fatty acid deficiency
Food/Nutrition History	Reports or observations of: ▪ Intake of essential fatty acids less than 10% of energy (primarily associated with PN)
Client History	▪ Conditions associated with a diagnosis or treatment, e.g., prolonged catabolic illness (e.g., AIDS, tuberculosis, anorexia nervosa, sepsis or severe infection from recent surgery) ▪ Severe fat malabsorption with bowel resection, pancreatic insufficiency, or hepatic disease accompanied by steatorrhea

Updated: 2008 Edition

INTAKE

EXCESSIVE FAT INTAKE (NI-5.6.2)

Definition
Higher fat intake compared to established reference standards or recommendations based on physiological needs.

Etiology (*Cause/Contributing Risk Factors*)
Factors gathered during the nutrition assessment process that contribute to the existence or the maintenance of pathophysiological, psychosocial, situational, developmental, cultural, and/or environmental problems:
- Food- and nutrition-related knowledge deficit
- Harmful beliefs/attitudes about food, nutrition, and nutrition-related topics
- Lack of access to healthful food choices, e.g., healthful food choices not provided as an option by caregiver or parent, homeless
- Changes in taste and appetite or preference
- Lack of value for behavior change, competing values

Signs/Symptoms (*Defining Characteristics*)
A typical cluster of subjective and objective signs and symptoms gathered during the nutrition assessment process that provide evidence that a problem exists; quantify the problem and describe its severity.

Nutrition Assessment Category	Potential Indicators of this Nutrition Diagnosis (one or more must be present)
Biochemical Data, Medical Tests and Procedures	▪ Cholesterol > 200 mg/dL (5.2 mmol/L), LDL cholesterol > 100 mg/dL (2.59 mmol/L), HDL cholesterol < 40 mg/dL (1.036 mmol/L), triglycerides > 150 mg/dL (1.695 mmol/L) ▪ Elevated serum amylase and/or lipase ▪ Elevated LFTs, T. Bili ▪ Fecal fat > 7g/24 hours
Anthropometric Measurements	
Physical Exam Findings	▪ Evidence of xanthomas

EXCESSIVE FAT INTAKE CONT'D (NI-5.6.2)

Food/Nutrition History	Reports or observations of: • Frequent or large portions of high-fat foods • Frequent food preparation with added fat • Frequent consumption of high risk lipids (i.e., saturated fat, trans fat, cholesterol) • Report of foods containing fat more than diet prescription
Client History	• Conditions associated with a diagnosis or treatment, e.g., hyperlipidemia, cystic fibrosis, angina, artherosclerosis, pancreatic, liver, and biliary diseases, post-transplantation • Medication, e.g., pancreatic enzymes, cholesterol- or other lipid-lowering medications • Diarrhea, cramping, steatorrhea, epigastric pain • Family history of hyperlipidemia, atherosclerosis, or pancreatitis

Updated: 2008 Edition

INAPPROPRIATE INTAKE OF FOOD FATS (SPECIFY) (NI-5.6.3)

Definition
Intake of wrong type or quality of food fats compared to established reference standards or recommendations based on physiological needs.

Etiology (*Cause/Contributing Risk Factors*)
Factors gathered during the nutrition assessment process that contribute to the existence or the maintenance of pathophysiological, psychosocial, situational, developmental, cultural, and/or environmental problems:
- Food- and nutrition-related knowledge deficit
- Harmful beliefs/attitudes about food, nutrition, and nutrition-related topics
- Lack of access to healthful food choices, e.g., healthful food choices not provided as an option by caregiver or parent, homeless
- Changes in taste and appetite or preference
- Lack of value for behavior change, competing values

Signs/Symptoms (*Defining Characteristics*)
A typical cluster of subjective and objective signs and symptoms gathered during the nutrition assessment process that provide evidence that a problem exists; quantify the problem and describe its severity.

Nutrition Assessment Category	Potential Indicators of this Nutrition Diagnosis (one or more must be present)
Biochemical Data, Medical Tests and Procedures	■ Cholesterol > 200 mg/dL (5.2 mmol/L), LDL cholesterol > 100 mg/dL (2.59 mmol/L), HDL cholesterol < 40 mg/dL (1.036 mmol/L), triglycerides > 150 mg/dL (1.695 mmol/L) ■ Elevated serum amylase and/or lipase ■ Elevated LFTs, T. Bili, C-reactive protein
Anthropometric Measurements	
Physical Exam Findings	■ Evidence of dermatitis
Food/Nutrition History	Reports or observations of: ■ Frequent food preparation with added fat that is not of desired type for condition ■ Frequent consumption of fats that are undesirable for condition (i.e., saturated fat, trans fat, cholesterol, Ω-6 fatty acids) ■ Inadequate intake of monounsaturated, polyunsaturated, or Ω-3 fatty acids
Client History	■ Conditions associated with a diagnosis or treatment of diabetes, cardiac diseases, obesity, liver or biliary disorders ■ Diarrhea, cramping, steatorrhea, epigastric pain ■ Family history of diabetes-related heart disease, hyperlipidemia, atherosclerosis, or pancreatitis

Updated: 2008 Edition

INADEQUATE PROTEIN INTAKE (NI-5.7.1)

Definition
Lower intake of protein-containing foods or substances compared to established reference standards or recommendations based on physiological needs.

Etiology (*Cause/Contributing Risk Factors*)
Factors gathered during the nutrition assessment process that contribute to the existence or the maintenance of pathophysiological, psychosocial, situational, developmental, cultural, and/or environmental problems:

- Physiological causes, e.g., increased nutrient needs due to prolonged catabolic illness, malabsorption, age, or condition
- Lack of access to food, e.g., economic constraints, cultural or religious practices, restricting food given to elderly and/or children
- Food- and nutrition-related knowledge deficit
- Psychological causes, e.g., depression or disordered eating

Signs/Symptoms (*Defining Characteristics*)
A typical cluster of subjective and objective signs and symptoms gathered during the nutrition assessment process that provide evidence that a problem exists; quantify the problem and describe its severity.

Nutrition Assessment Category	Potential Indicators of this Nutrition Diagnosis (one or more must be present)
Biochemical Data, Medical Tests and Procedures	
Anthropometric Measurements	
Physical Examination Findings	
Food/Nutrition History	Reports or observation of: ■ Insufficient intake of protein to meet requirements ■ Cultural or religious practices that limit protein intake ■ Economic constraints that limit food availability ■ Prolonged adherence to a very–low-protein weight-loss diet
Client History	■ Conditions associated with a diagnosis or treatment, e.g., severe protein malabsorption such as bowel resection

EXCESSIVE PROTEIN INTAKE (NI-5.7.2)

Definition
Intake more than the recommended level of protein compared to established reference standards or recommendations based on physiological needs.

Etiology (*Cause/Contributing Risk Factors*)
Factors gathered during the nutrition assessment process that contribute to the existence or the maintenance of pathophysiological, psychosocial, situational, developmental, cultural, and/or environmental problems:
- Liver dysfunction
- Renal dysfunction
- Harmful beliefs/attitudes about food, nutrition, and nutrition-related topics
- Lack of access to specialized protein products
- Metabolic abnormality
- Food faddism

Signs/Symptoms (*Defining Characteristics*)
A typical cluster of subjective and objective signs and symptoms gathered during the nutrition assessment process that provide evidence that a problem exists; quantify the problem and describe its severity.

Nutrition Assessment Category	Potential Indicators of this Nutrition Diagnosis (one or more must be present)
Biochemical Data, Medical Tests and Procedures	▪ Altered laboratory values, e.g., ↑ BUN, ↓ glomerular filtration rate (altered renal status)
Anthropometric Measurements	▪ Growth stunting or failure based on National Center for Health Statistics growth charts (metabolic disorders)
Physical Exam Findings	
Food/Nutrition History	Reports or observations of: ▪ Higher than recommended total protein intake, e.g., early renal disease, advanced liver disease with confusion ▪ Inappropriate supplementation
Client History	▪ Conditions associated with a diagnosis or treatment, e.g., early renal disease or advanced liver disease with confusion

Edition: 2008

INAPPROPRIATE
INTAKE OF AMINO ACIDS (SPECIFY) (NI-5.7.3)

Definition
Intake that is more or less than recommended level and/or type of amino acids compared to established reference standards or recommendations based on physiological needs.

Etiology (*Cause/Contributing Risk Factors*)
Factors gathered during the nutrition assessment process that contribute to the existence or the maintenance of pathophysiological, psychosocial, situational, developmental, cultural, and/or environmental problems:

- Liver dysfunction
- Renal dysfunction
- Harmful beliefs/attitudes about food, nutrition, and nutrition-related topics
- Misused specialized protein products
- Metabolic abnormality
- Food faddism
- Inborn errors of metabolism

SIGNS/SYMPTOMS (*Defining Characteristics*)
A typical cluster of subjective and objective signs and symptoms gathered during the nutrition assessment process that provide evidence that a problem exists; quantify the problem and describe its severity.

Nutrition Assessment Category	Potential Indicators of this Nutrition Diagnosis (one or more must be present)
Biochemical Data, Medical Tests and Procedures	▪ Altered laboratory values, e.g., ↑ BUN, ↓ glomerular filtration rate (altered renal status); increased urinary 3-methyl-histidine ▪ Elevated specific amino acids (inborn errors of metabolism) ▪ Elevated homocysteine or ammonia
Anthropometric Measurements	
Physical Exam Findings	▪ Physical or neurological changes (inborn errors of metabolism)

INAPPROPRIATE
INTAKE OF AMINO ACIDS (SPECIFY) (NI-5.7.3)

Food/Nutrition History	Reports or observation of: ▪ Higher than recommended amino acid intake, e.g., early renal disease, advanced liver disease, inborn error of metabolism ▪ Higher than recommended type of amino acids for prescribed parenteral and enteral nutrition therapy ▪ Inappropriate amino acid or protein supplementation, as for athletes ▪ Higher than recommended amino acid intake, e.g., excess phenylalanine intake
Client History	▪ Conditions associated with a diagnosis or treatment of illness that requires PEN therapy ▪ History of inborn error of metabolism ▪ Uremia, azotemia (renal patients)

INTAKE

Edition: 2008

INADEQUATE CARBOHYDRATE INTAKE (NI-5.8.1)

Definition

Lower intake of carbohydrate-containing foods or substances compared to established reference standards or recommendations based on physiological needs.

Etiology (*Cause/Contributing Risk Factors*)

Factors gathered during the nutrition assessment process that contribute to the existence or the maintenance of pathophysiological, psychosocial, situational, developmental, cultural, and/or environmental problems:

- Physiological causes, e.g., increased energy needs due to increased activity level or metabolic change, malabsorption
- Lack of access to food, e.g., economic constraints, cultural or religious practices, restricting food given to elderly and/or children
- Food- and nutrition-related knowledge deficit
- Psychological causes, e.g., depression or disordered eating

Signs/Symptoms (*Defining Characteristics*)

A typical cluster of subjective and objective signs and symptoms gathered during the nutrition assessment process that provide evidence that a problem exists; quantify the problem and describe its severity.

Nutrition Assessment Category	Potential Indicators of this Nutrition Diagnosis (one or more must be present)
Biochemical Data, Medical Tests and Procedures	
Anthropometric Measurements	
Physical Examination Findings	▪ Ketone smell on breath
Food/Nutrition History	Reports or observation of: ▪ Carbohydrate intake less than recommended amounts ▪ Inability to independently consume foods/fluids, e.g., diminished mobility in hand, wrist, or digits
Client History	▪ Conditions associated with a diagnosis or treatment, e.g., pancreatic insufficiency, hepatic disease, celiac disease, seizure disorder, or carbohydrate malabsorption

EXCESSIVE CARBOHYDRATE INTAKE (NI-5.8.2)

Definition

Intake more than the recommended level and type of carbohydrate compared to established reference standards or recommendations based on physiological needs.

Etiology (*Cause/Contributing Risk Factors*)

Factors gathered during the nutrition assessment process that contribute to the existence or the maintenance of pathophysiological, psychosocial, situational, developmental, cultural, and/or environmental problems:

- Physiological causes requiring modified carbohydrate intake, e.g., diabetes mellitus, lactase deficiency, sucrase-isomaltase deficiency, aldolase-B deficiency
- Cultural or religious practices that interfere with the ability to reduce carbohydrate intake
- Food- and nutrition-related knowledge deficit, e.g., inability to access sufficient information concerning appropriate carbohydrate intake
- Food and nutrition compliance limitations, e.g., lack of willingness or failure to modify carbohydrate intake in response to recommendations from a dietitian or physician
- Psychological causes, e.g., depression or disordered eating

Signs/Symptoms (*Defining Characteristics*)

A typical cluster of subjective and objective signs and symptoms gathered during the nutrition assessment process that provide evidence that a problem exists; quantify the problem and describe its severity.

Nutrition Assessment Category	Potential Indicators of this Nutrition Diagnosis (one or more must be present)
Biochemical Data, Medical Tests and Procedures	▪ Hyperglycemia (fasting blood sugar > 126 mg/dL) ▪ Hemoglobin A1C > 6% ▪ Abnormal oral glucose tolerance test (2-hour post load glucose > 200 mg/dL)
Anthropometric Measurements	
Physical Examination Findings	▪ Dental caries ▪ Diarrhea in response to carbohydrate feeding

Edition: 2008

EXCESSIVE CARBOHYDRATE INTAKE CONT'D (NI-5.8.2)

Food/Nutrition History	Reports or observation of: • Cultural or religious practices that do not support modification of dietary carbohydrate intake • Economic constraints that limit availability of appropriate foods • Carbohydrate intake that is consistently more than recommended amounts
Client History	• Conditions associated with a diagnosis or treatment of, e.g., diabetes mellitus, inborn errors of carbohydrate metabolism, lactase deficiency, severe infection, sepsis, or obesity • Chronic use of medications that cause hyperglycemia, e.g., steroids • Pancreatic insufficiency resulting in reduced insulin production

INAPPROPRIATE
INTAKE OF TYPES OF CARBOHYDRATES (SPECIFY) (NI-5.8.3)

Definition

Intake of the type or amount of carbohydrate that is more or less than the established reference standards or recommendations based on physiological needs.

Etiology (*Cause/Contributing Risk Factors*)

Factors gathered during the nutrition assessment process that contribute to the existence or the maintenance of pathophysiological, psychosocial, situational, developmental, cultural, and/or environmental problems:

- Physiological causes requiring careful use of modified carbohydrate, e.g., diabetes mellitus, metabolic syndrome, hypoglycemia, celiac disease, allergies, obesity
- Cultural or religious practices that interfere with the ability to regulate types of carbohydrate consumed
- Food- and nutrition-related knowledge deficit, e.g., inability to access sufficient information concerning more appropriate carbohydrate types and/or amounts
- Food and nutrition compliance limitations, e.g., lack of willingness or failure to modify carbohydrate intake in response to recommendations from a dietitian, physician, or caregiver
- Psychological causes, e.g., depression or disordered eating

Signs/Symptoms (*Defining Characteristics*)

A typical cluster of subjective and objective signs and symptoms gathered during the nutrition assessment process that provide evidence that a problem exists; quantify the problem and describe its severity.

Nutrition Assessment Category	Potential Indicators of this Nutrition Diagnosis (one or more must be present)
Biochemical Data, Medical Tests and Procedures	• Hypoglycemia or hyperglycemia documented on regular basis when compared with goal of maintaining glucose levels at or less than 140 mg/dL throughout the day
Anthropometric Measurements	
Physical Examination Findings	

Edition: 2008

INAPPROPRIATE INTAKE OF TYPES OF CARBOHYDRATES (SPECIFY) CONT'D (NI-5.8.3)

Food/Nutrition History	Reports or observations of: • Diarrhea in response to high intake of refined carbohydrates • Economic constraints that limit availability of appropriate foods • Carbohydrate intake that is different from recommended types • Allergic reactions to certain carbohydrate foods or food groups • Limited knowledge of carbohydrate composition of foods or of carbohydrate metabolism
Client History	• Conditions associated with a diagnosis or treatment, e.g., diabetes mellitus, obesity, metabolic syndrome, hypoglycemia • Chronic use of medications that cause altered glucose levels, e.g., steroids, antidepressants, antipsychotics

INTAKE

INCONSISTENT CARBOHYDRATE INTAKE (NI-5.8.4)

Definition
Inconsistent timing of carbohydrate intake throughout the day, day to day, or a pattern of carbohydrate intake that is not consistent with recommended pattern based on physiological or medication needs.

Etiology (*Cause/Contributing Risk Factors*)
Factors gathered during the nutrition assessment process that contribute to the existence or the maintenance of pathophysiological, psychosocial, situational, developmental, cultural, and/or environmental problems:

* Physiological causes requiring careful timing and consistency in the amount of carbohydrate, e.g., diabetes mellitus, hypoglycemia
* Cultural or religious practices or lifestyle factors that interfere with the ability to regulate timing of carbohydrate consumption
* Food- and nutrition-related knowledge deficit, e.g., inability to access sufficient information concerning more appropriate timing of carbohydrate intake
* Food and nutrition compliance limitations, e.g., lack of willingness or failure to modify carbohydrate timing in response to recommendations from a dietitian, physician, or caregiver
* Psychological causes, e.g., depression or disordered eating

Signs/Symptoms (*Defining Characteristics*)
A typical cluster of subjective and objective signs and symptoms gathered during the nutrition assessment process that provide evidence that a problem exists; quantify the problem and describe its severity.

Nutrition Assessment Category	Potential Indicators of this Nutrition Diagnosis (one or more must be present)
Biochemical Data, Medical Tests and Procedures	▪ Hypoglycemia or hyperglycemia documented on regular basis associated with inconsistent carbohydrate intake ▪ Wide variations in blood glucose levels
Anthropometric Measurements	
Physical Examination Findings	
Food/Nutrition History	Reports or observations of: ▪ Economic constraints that limit availability of appropriate foods ▪ Carbohydrate intake that is different from recommended types or ingested on an irregular basis
Client History	▪ Conditions associated with a diagnosis or treatment, e.g., diabetes mellitus, obesity, metabolic syndrome, hypoglycemia ▪ Use of insulin or insulin secretagogues ▪ Chronic use of medications that cause altered glucose levels, e.g., steroids, antidepressants, antipsychotics

INTAKE

Edition: 2008

INADEQUATE FIBER INTAKE (NI-5.8.5)

Definition
Lower intake of fiber-containing foods or substances compared to established reference standards or recommendations based on physiological needs.

Etiology (*Cause/Contributing Risk Factors*)
Factors gathered during the nutrition assessment process that contribute to the existence or the maintenance of pathophysiological, psychosocial, situational, developmental, cultural, and/or environmental problems:

- Lack of access to fiber-containing foods
- Food- and nutrition-related knowledge deficit
- Psychological causes, e.g., depression or disordered eating
- Prolonged adherence to a low-fiber or low-residue diet
- Difficulty chewing or swallowing high-fiber foods
- Economic constraints that limit availability of appropriate foods
- Inability or unwillingness to purchase or consume fiber-containing foods
- Inappropriate food preparation practices, e.g., reliance on overprocessed, overcooked foods

Signs/Symptoms (*Defining Characteristics*)
A typical cluster of subjective and objective signs and symptoms gathered during the nutrition assessment process that provide evidence that a problem exists; quantify the problem and describe its severity.

Nutrition Assessment Category	Potential Indicators of this Nutrition Diagnosis (one or more must be present)
Biochemical Data, Medical Tests and Procedures	
Anthropometric Measurements	
Physical Examination Findings	
Food/Nutrition History	Reports or observations of: ▪ Insufficient intake of fiber when compared to recommended amounts (38 g/day for men and 25 g/day for women)
Client History	▪ Conditions associated with a diagnosis or treatment, e.g., ulcer disease, inflammatory bowel disease, or short-bowel syndrome treated with a low-fiber diet ▪ Low stool volume, constipation

Updated: 2008 Edition

INTAKE

EXCESSIVE FIBER INTAKE (NI-5.8.6)

Definition
Higher intake of fiber-containing foods or substances compared to recommendations based on patient/client condition.

Etiology (*Cause/Contributing Risk Factors*)
Factors gathered during the nutrition assessment process that contribute to the existence or the maintenance of pathophysiological, psychosocial, situational, developmental, cultural, and/or environmental problems:

- Food- and nutrition-related knowledge deficit about desirable quantities of fiber for individual condition
- Harmful beliefs or attitudes about food- or nutrition-related topics, e.g., obsession with bowel frequency and habits
- Lack of knowledge about appropriate fiber intake for condition
- Food preparation or eating patterns that involve only high-fiber foods to the exclusion of other nutrient-dense foods

Signs/Symptoms (*Defining Characteristics*)
A typical cluster of subjective and objective signs and symptoms gathered during the nutrition assessment process that provide evidence that a problem exists; quantify the problem and describe its severity.

Nutrition Assessment Category	Potential Indicators of this Nutrition Diagnosis (one or more must be present)
Biochemical Data, Medical Tests and Procedures	
Anthropometric Measurements	
Physical Examination Findings	
Food/Nutrition History	Reports or observations of: ▪ Fiber intake higher than tolerated or generally recommended for current medical condition
Client History	▪ Conditions associated with a diagnosis or treatment, e.g., ulcer disease, irritable bowel syndrome, inflammatory bowel disease, short-bowel syndrome, diverticulitis, obstructive constipation, prolapsing hemorrhoids, gastrointestinal stricture, eating disorders, or mental illness with obsessive-compulsive tendencies ▪ Nausea, vomiting, excessive flatulence, diarrhea, abdominal cramping, high stool volume or frequency that causes discomfort to the individual; obstruction; phytobezoar

Updated: 2008 Edition

INADEQUATE VITAMIN INTAKE (SPECIFY) (NI-5.9.1)

Definition

Lower intake of vitamin-containing foods or substances compared to established reference standards or recommendations based on physiological needs.

Etiology (*Cause/Contributing Risk Factors*)

Factors gathered during the nutrition assessment process that contribute to the existence or the maintenance of pathophysiological, psychosocial, situational, developmental, cultural, and/or environmental problems:

- Physiological causes, e.g., increased nutrient needs due to prolonged catabolic illness, disease state, malabsorption, or medications
- Lack of access to food, e.g., economic constraints, cultural or religious practices, restricting food given to elderly and/or children
- Food- and nutrition-related knowledge deficit concerning food sources of vitamins
- Psychological causes, e.g., depression or eating disorders

Signs/Symptoms (*Defining Characteristics*)

A typical cluster of subjective and objective signs and symptoms gathered during the nutrition assessment process that provide evidence that a problem exists; quantify the problem and describe its severity.

Nutrition Assessment Category	Potential Indicators of this Nutrition Diagnosis (one or more must be present)
Biochemical Data, Medical Tests and Procedures	▪ Vitamin A: serum retinol < 10 µg/dL (0.35 µmol/L)
	▪ Vitamin C: plasma concentrations < 0.2 mg/dL (11.4 µmol/L)
	▪ Vitamin D: ionized calcium < 3.9 mg/dL (0.98 mmol/L) with elevated parathyroid hormone, normal serum calcium, and serum phosphorus < 2.6 mg/dL (0.84 mmol/L)
	▪ Vitamin E: plasma alpha-tocopherol < 18 µmol/g (41.8 µmol/L)
	▪ Vitamin K: elevated prothrombin time; altered INR (without anticoagulation therapy)
	▪ Thiamin: erythrocyte transketolase activity > 1.20 µg/mL/h
	▪ Riboflavin: erythrocyte glutathione reductase > 1.2 IU/g hemoglobin
	▪ Niacin: N'methyl-nicotinamide excretion < 5.8 µmol/day
	▪ Vitamin B-6: plasma pryrdoxal 5'phosphate < 5 ng/mL (20 nmol/L)
	▪ Vitamin B-12: serum concentration < 24.4 ng/dL (180 pmol/L); elevated homocysteine
	▪ Folic acid—serum concentration < 0.3 µg/dL (7 nmol/L); red cell folate < 315 nmol/L

INADEQUATE VITAMIN INTAKE (SPECIFY) (NI-5.9.1)

Anthropometric Measurements	
Physical Exam Findings	▪ Vitamin A: night blindness, Bitot's spots, xerophthalmia, follicular hyperkeratosis ▪ Vitamin C: follicular hyperkeratosis, petichiae, ecchymosis, coiled hairs, inflamed and bleeding gums, perifolicular hemorrhages, joint effusions, arthralgia, and impaired wound healing ▪ Vitamin D: widening at ends of long bones ▪ Riboflavin: sore throat, hyperemia, edema of pharyngeal and oral mucous membranes, cheilosis, angular stomatitis, glossitis, magenta tongue, seborrheic dermatitis, and normochromic, normocytic anemia with pure erythrocyte cytoplasia of the bone marrow ▪ Niacin: symmetrical, pigmented rash on areas exposed to sunlight; bright red tongue ▪ Vitamin B-6: seborrheic dermatitis, stomatitis, cheilosis, glossitis, confusion, depression ▪ Vitamin B-12: tingling and numbness in extremities, diminished vibratory and position sense, motor disturbances including gait disturbances
Food/Nutrition History	Reports or observations of: ▪ Dietary history reflects inadequate intake of foods containing specific vitamins as compared to requirements or recommended level ▪ Dietary history reflects excessive consumption of foods that do not contain available vitamins, e.g., over processed, overcooked, or improperly stored foods ▪ Prolonged use of substances known to increase vitamin requirements or reduce vitamin absorption ▪ Lack of interest in foods ▪ Vitamin/mineral deficiency
Client History	▪ Conditions associated with a diagnosis or treatment, e.g., malabsorption as a result of celiac disease, short-bowel syndrome, or inflammatory bowel ▪ Certain environmental conditions, e.g., infants exclusively fed breast milk with limited exposure to sunlight (Vitamin D) ▪ Rachitic rosary in children, rickets, osteomalacia ▪ Pellegra

INTAKE

Edition: 2008

EXCESSIVE VITAMIN INTAKE (SPECIFY) (NI-5.9.2)

Definition

Higher intake of vitamin-containing foods or substances compared to established reference standards or recommendations based on physiological needs.

Etiology (*Cause/Contributing Risk Factors*)

Factors gathered during the nutrition assessment process that contribute to the existence or the maintenance of pathophysiological, psychosocial, situational, developmental, cultural, and/or environmental problems:

- Physiological causes, e.g., decreased nutrient needs due to prolonged immobility or chronic renal disease
- Access to foods and supplements in excess of needs, e.g., cultural or religious practices, inappropriate food and supplements given to pregnant women, elderly, or children
- Food- and nutrition-related knowledge deficit concerning food and supplemental sources of vitamins
- Psychological causes, e.g., depression or eating disorders
- Accidental overdose from oral and supplemental forms, enteral or parenteral sources

Signs/Symptoms (*Defining Characteristics*)

A typical cluster of subjective and objective signs and symptoms gathered during the nutrition assessment process that provide evidence that a problem exists; quantify the problem and describe its severity.

Nutrition Assessment Category	Potential Indicators of this Nutrition Diagnosis (one or more must be present)
Biochemical Data, Medical Tests and Procedures	▪ Vitamin D: ionized calcium > 5.4 mg/dL (1.35 mmol/L) with elevated parathyroid hormone, normal serum calcium, and serum phosphorus > 2.6 mg/dL (0.84 mmol/L) ▪ Vitamin K: slowed prothrombin time or altered INR ▪ Niacin: N'methyl-nicotinamide excretion > 7.3 µmol/day ▪ Vitamin B-6: plasma pryrdoxal 5'phosphate > 15.7 ng/mL (94 noml/L) ▪ Vitamin A: serum retinol concentration > 60 µg/dL (2.09 µmol/L)
Anthropometric Measurements	▪ Vitamin D: growth retardation

EXCESSIVE VITAMIN INTAKE (SPECIFY) (NI-5.9.2)

Physical Exam Findings	• Vitamin A: changes in the skin and mucous membranes; dry lips (cheilitis); early—dryness of the nasal mucosa and eyes; later—dryness, erythema, scaling and peeling of the skin, hair loss, and nail fragility. Headache, nausea, and vomiting. Infants may have bulging fontanelle; children may develop bone alterations. • Vitamin D: elevated serum calcium (hypercalcemia) and phosphorus (hyperphosphatemia) levels; calcification of soft tissues (calcinosis), including the kidney, lungs, heart, and even the tympanic membrane of the ear, which can result in deafness. Headache and nausea. Infants given excessive amounts of vitamin D may have gastrointestinal upset, bone fragility. • Vitamin K: hemolytic anemia in adults or severe jaundice in infants have been noted on rare occasions • Niacin: histamine release, which causes flushing, aggravation of asthma, or liver disease
Food/Nutrition History	Reports or observations of: • History or measured intake reflects excessive intake of foods and supplements containing vitamins as compared to estimated requirements, including fortified cereals, meal replacements, vitamin-mineral supplements, other dietary supplements (e.g., fish liver oils or capsules), tube feeding, and/or parenteral solutions • Intake > Tolerable Upper Limit (UL) for vitamin A (as retinol ester, not as ᴅ-carotene) is 600 µg/d for infants and toddlers; 900 µg/d for children 4-8 y, 1700 µg/d for children 9-13 y, 2800 for children 14-18 y, and 3000 µg/d for adults • Intake more than UL for vitamin D is 25 µg/d for infants and 50 µg/d for children and adults • Niacin: clinical, high-dose niacinamide (NA), 1-2 g, three times per day, can have side effects
Client History	• Conditions associated with a diagnosis or treatment, e.g., chronic liver or kidney diseases, heart failure, cancer

Edition: 2008

INADEQUATE MINERAL INTAKE (SPECIFY) (NI-5.10.1)

Definition

Lower intake of mineral-containing foods or substances compared to established reference standards or recommendations based on physiological needs.

Etiology (*Cause/Contributing Risk Factors*)

Factors gathered during the nutrition assessment process that contribute to the existence or the maintenance of pathophysiological, psychosocial, situational, developmental, cultural, and/or environmental problems:

- Physiological causes, e.g., increased nutrient needs due to prolonged catabolic illness, malabsorption, hyperexcretion, nutrient/drug and nutrient/nutrient interaction, growth and maturation
- Lack of access to food, e.g., economic constraints, cultural or religious practices, restricting food given to elderly and/or children
- Food- and nutrition-related knowledge deficit concerning food sources of minerals; misdiagnosis of lactose intolerance/lactase deficiency; perception of conflicting nutrition messages from health professionals; inappropriate reliance on supplements
- Psychological causes, e.g., depression or eating disorders
- Environmental causes, e.g., inadequately tested nutrient bioavailability of fortified foods, beverages, and supplements; inappropriate marketing of fortified foods/beverages/supplements as a substitute for natural food source of nutrient(s)

Signs/Symptoms (*Defining Characteristics*)

A typical cluster of subjective and objective signs and symptoms gathered during the nutrition assessment process that provide evidence that a problem exists; quantify the problem and describe its severity.

Nutrition Assessment Category	Potential Indicators of this Nutrition Diagnosis (one or more must be present)
Biochemical Data, Medical Tests and Procedures	▪ Calcium: bone mineral content (BMC) below the young adult mean. Hypocalciuria, serum 25(OH)D < 32 ng/mL ▪ Phosphorus < 2.6 mg/dL (0.84 mmol/L) ▪ Magnesium < 1.8 mg/dL (0.7 mmol/L) ▪ Iron: hemoglobin < 13 g/L (2 mmol/L) (males); < 12 g/L (1.86 mmol/L) (females) ▪ Iodine: urinary excretion < 100 µg/L (788 nmol/L) ▪ Copper, serum copper < 64 µg/dL (10 µmol/L)
Anthropometric Measurements	▪ Height loss
Physical Exam Findings	▪ Calcium: diminished bone mineral density, hypertension, obesity

INADEQUATE MINERAL INTAKE (SPECIFY) (NI-5.10.1)

Food/Nutrition History	Reports or observations of insufficient mineral intake from diet compared to recommended intake: ▪ Food avoidance and/or elimination of whole food group(s) from diet ▪ Lack of interest in food ▪ Inappropriate food choices and/or chronic dieting behavior ▪ Vitamin/mineral deficiency
Client History	▪ Conditions associated with a diagnosis or treatment, e.g., malabsorption as a result of celiac disease, short bowel syndrome, inflammatory bowel disease, or post-menopausal women without estrogen supplementation and increased calcium need ▪ Polycystic ovary syndrome, premenstrual syndrome, kidney stones, colon polyps ▪ Other significant medical diagnoses and therapies ▪ Geographic latitude and history of Ultraviolet-B exposure/use of sunscreen ▪ Change in living environment/independence

Updated: Edition 2008

INTAKE

EXCESSIVE MINERAL INTAKE (SPECIFY) (NI-5.10.2)

Definition

Higher intake of mineral from foods, supplements, medications or water, compared to established reference standards or recommendations based on physiological needs.

Etiology (*Cause/Contributing Risk Factors*)

Factors gathered during the nutrition assessment process that contribute to the existence or the maintenance of pathophysiological, psychosocial, situational, developmental, cultural, and/or environmental problems:

- Food- and nutrition-related knowledge deficit
- Harmful beliefs/attitudes about food, nutrition, and nutrition-related topics
- Food faddism
- Accidental oversupplementation
- Overconsumption of a limited variety of foods
- Lack of knowledge about management of diagnosed genetic disorder altering mineral homeostasis [hemochromatosis (iron), Wilson's disease (copper)]
- Lack of knowledge about management of diagnosed disease state requiring mineral restriction [cholestatic liver disease (copper and manganese), renal insufficiency (phosphorus, magnesium, potassium)]

Signs/Symptoms (*Defining Characteristics*)

A typical cluster of subjective and objective signs and symptoms gathered during the nutrition assessment process that provide evidence that a problem exists; quantify the problem and describe its severity.

Nutrition Assessment Category	Potential Indicators of this Nutrition Diagnosis (one or more must be present)
Biochemical Data, Medical Tests and Procedures	Changes in appropriate laboratory values, such as: • ↑ TSH (iodine supplementation) • ↓ HDL (zinc supplementation) • ↑ Serum ferritin and transferrin saturation (iron overload) • Hyperphosphatemia • Hypermagnesemia
Anthropometric Measurements	
Physical Exam Findings	• Hair and nail changes (selenium)
Food/Nutrition History	Reports or observations of: • High intake of foods or supplements containing mineral compared to DRIs • Anorexia (zinc supplementation)
Client History	• GI disturbances (iron, magnesium, copper, zinc, selenium) • Copper deficiency anemia (zinc) • Liver damage (copper, iron), enamel or skeletal fluorosis (fluoride)

SWALLOWING DIFFICULTY (NC-1.1)

Definition
Impaired or difficult movement of food and liquid within the oral cavity to the stomach

Etiology (*Cause/Contributing Risk Factors*)
Factors gathered during the nutrition assessment process that contribute to the existence or the maintenance of pathophysiological, psychosocial, situational, developmental, cultural, and/or environmental problems:
- Mechanical causes, e.g., inflammation, surgery, stricture, or oral, pharyngeal and esophageal tumors, mechanical ventilation
- Motor causes, e.g., neurological or muscular disorders, such as, cerebral palsy, stroke, multiple sclerosis, scleroderma, prematurity

Signs/Symptoms (*Defining Characteristics*)
A typical cluster of subjective and objective signs and symptoms gathered during the nutrition assessment process that provide evidence that a problem exists; quantify the problem and describe its severity.

Nutrition Assessment Category	Potential Indicators of this Nutrition Diagnosis (one or more must be present)
Biochemical Data, Medical Tests and Procedures	▪ Radiological findings, e.g., abnormal swallowing studies
Anthropometric Measurements	
Physical Exam Findings	▪ Evidence of dehydration, e.g., dry mucous membranes, poor skin turgor ▪ Non-normal findings in cranial nerves and (CN VII) muscles of facial expression, (Nerve IX) gag reflex, swallow (Nerve X) and tongue range of motions (Nerve XII), cough reflex, drooling, facial weakness and ability to perform and wet and dry swallow
Food/Nutrition History	Reports or observations of: ▪ Coughing, choking, prolonged chewing, pouching of food, regurgitation, facial expression changes during eating, prolonged feeding time, drooling, noisy wet upper airway sounds, feeling of "food getting stuck," pain while swallowing ▪ Decreased food intake ▪ Avoidance of foods ▪ Mealtime resistance
Client History	▪ Conditions associated with a diagnosis or treatment, e.g., dysphagia, achalasia ▪ Repeated upper respiratory infections and or pneumonia

Updated: 2008 Edition

BITING/CHEWING (MASTICATORY) DIFFICULTY (NC-1.2)

Definition
Impaired ability to bite or chew food in preparation for swallowing.

Etiology (Cause/Contributing Risk Factors)
Factors gathered during the nutrition assessment process that contribute to the existence or the maintenance of pathophysiological, psychosocial, situational, developmental, cultural, and/or environmental problems:

- Craniofacial malformations
- Oral surgery
- Neuromuscular dysfunction
- Partial or complete edentulism
- Soft tissue disease (primary or oral manifestations of a systemic disease)
- Xerostomia

Signs/Symptoms (Defining Characteristics)
A typical cluster of subjective and objective signs and symptoms gathered during the nutrition assessment process that provide evidence that a problem exists; quantify the problem and describe its severity.

Nutrition Assessment Category	Potential Indicators of this Nutrition Diagnosis (one or more must be present)
Biochemical Data, Medical Tests and Procedures	
Anthropometric Measurements	
Physical Exam Findings	▪ Partial or complete edentulism ▪ Alterations in cranial nerve function (V, VII, IX, X, XII) ▪ Dry mouth ▪ Oral lesions interfering with eating ability ▪ Impaired tongue movement ▪ Ill-fitting dentures or broken dentures

BITING/CHEWING (MASTICATORY) DIFFICULTY (NC-1.2)

Food/Nutrition History	Reports or observations of: • Decreased intake of food • Alterations in food intake from usual • Decreased intake or avoidance of food difficult to form into a bolus, e.g., nuts, whole pieces of meat, poultry, fish, fruits, vegetables • Avoidance of foods of age-appropriate texture • Spitting food out or prolonged feeding time
Client History	• Conditions associated with a diagnosis or treatment, e.g., alcoholism; Alzheimer's; head, neck or pharyngeal cancer; cerebral palsy; cleft lip/palate; oral soft tissue infections (e.g., candidiasis, leukoplakia); lack of developmental readiness; oral manifestations of systemic disease (e.g., rheumatoid arthritis, lupus, Crohn's disease, penphigus vulgaris, HIV, diabetes) • Recent major oral surgery • Wired jaw • Chemotherapy with oral side effects • Radiation therapy to oral cavity

Updated: 2008 Edition

CLINICAL

BREASTFEEDING DIFFICULTY (NC-1.3)

Definition
Inability to sustain infant nutrition through breastfeeding.

Etiology (*Cause/Contributing Risk Factors*)
Factors gathered during the nutrition assessment process that contribute to the existence or the maintenance of pathophysiological, psychosocial, situational, developmental, cultural, and/or environmental problems:

Infant:

- Difficulty latching on, e.g., tight frenulum
- Poor sucking ability
- Oral pain
- Malnutrition/malabsorption
- Lethargy, sleepiness
- Irritability
- Swallowing difficulty

Mother:

- Painful breasts, nipples
- Breast or nipple abnormality
- Mastitis
- Perception of inadequate milk supply
- Lack of social, cultural, or environmental support

Signs/Symptoms (*Defining Characteristics*)
A typical cluster of subjective and objective signs and symptoms gathered during the nutrition assessment process that provide evidence that a problem exists; quantify the problem and describe its severity.

Nutrition Assessment Category	Potential Indicators of this Nutrition Diagnosis (one or more must be present)
Biochemical Data, Medical Tests and Procedures	▪ Laboratory evidence of dehydration (infant)
Anthropometric Measurements	▪ Any weight loss or poor weight gain (infant)
Physical Exam Findings	▪ Frenulum abnormality (infant) ▪ Vomiting or diarrhea (infant)

BREASTFEEDING DIFFICULTY (NC-1.3)

Food/Nutrition History	Reports or observations of (infant): • Coughing • Crying, latching on and off, pounding on breasts • Decreased feeding frequency/duration, early cessation of feeding, and/or feeding resistance • Lethargy • Hunger, lack of satiety after feeding • Fewer than six wet diapers in 24 hours Reports or observations of (mother): • Small amount of milk when pumping • Lack of confidence in ability to breastfeed • Doesn't hear infant swallowing • Concerns regarding mother's choice to breastfeed/lack of support • Insufficient knowledge of breastfeeding or infant hunger/satiety signals • Lack of facilities or accommodations at place of employment or in community for breastfeeding
Client History	• Conditions associated with a diagnosis or treatment of (infant), e.g., cleft lip/palate, thrush, premature birth, malabsorption, infection • Conditions associated with a diagnosis or treatment of (mother), e.g., mastitis, candidiasis, engorgement, history of breast surgery

CLINICAL

    Edition: 2008

ALTERED GASTROINTESTINAL (GI) FUNCTION (NC-1.4)

Definition
Changes in ability to digest or absorb nutrients.

Etiology (*Cause/Contributing Risk Factors*)
Factors gathered during the nutrition assessment process that contribute to the existence or the maintenance of pathophysiological, psychosocial, situational, developmental, cultural, and/or environmental problems:

- Alterations in GI anatomical structure, e.g., gastric bypass, Roux En Y
- Changes in the GI tract motility, e.g., gastroparesis
- Compromised GI tract function, e.g., celiac disease, Crohn's disease, infection, radiation therapy
- Compromised function of related GI organs, e.g., pancreas, liver
- Decreased functional length of the GI tract, e.g., short-bowel syndrome

Signs/Symptoms (*Defining Characteristics*)
A typical cluster of subjective and objective signs and symptoms gathered during the nutrition assessment process that provide evidence that a problem exists; quantify the problem and describe its severity.

Nutrition Assessment Category	Potential Indicators of this Nutrition Diagnosis (one or more must be present)
Biochemical Data, Medical Tests and Procedures	▪ Abnormal digestive enzyme and fecal fat studies ▪ Abnormal hydrogen breath test, d-xylose test, stool culture, and gastric emptying and/or small bowel transit time ▪ Endoscopic or colonoscopic examination results, biopsy results
Anthropometric Measurements	▪ Wasting due to malnutrition in severe cases
Physical Exam Findings	▪ Abdominal distension ▪ Increased (or sometimes decreased) bowel sounds
Food/Nutrition History	Reports or observations of: ▪ Avoidance or limitation of total intake or intake of specific foods/food groups due to GI symptoms, e.g., bloating, cramping, pain, diarrhea, steatorrhea (greasy, floating, foul-smelling stools) especially following ingestion of food
Client History	▪ Anorexia, nausea, vomiting, diarrhea, steatorrhea, constipation, abdominal pain ▪ Conditions associated with a diagnosis or treatment, e.g., malabsorption, maldigestion, steatorrhea, constipation, diverticulitis, Crohn's disease, inflammatory bowel disease, cystic fibrosis, celiac disease, irritable bowel syndrome, infection ▪ Surgical procedures, e.g., esophagectomy, dilatation, gastrectomy, vagotomy, gastric bypass, bowel resections

Updated: 2008 Edition

IMPAIRED NUTRIENT UTILIZATION (NC-2.1)

Definition
Changes in ability to absorb or metabolize nutrients and bioactive substances.

Etiology (*Cause/Contributing Risk Factors*)
Factors gathered during the nutrition assessment process that contribute to the existence or the maintenance of pathophysiological, psychosocial, situational, developmental, cultural, and/or environmental problems:
- Alterations in gastrointestinal anatomical structure
- Compromised function of the GI tract
- Compromised function of related GI organs, e.g., pancreas, liver
- Decreased functional length of the GI tract
- Metabolic disorders

Signs/Symptoms (*Defining Characteristics*)
A typical cluster of subjective and objective signs and symptoms gathered during the nutrition assessment process that provide evidence that a problem exists; quantify the problem and describe its severity.

Nutrition Assessment Category	Potential Indicators of this Nutrition Diagnosis (one or more must be present)
Biochemical Data, Medical Tests and Procedures	▪ Abnormal digestive enzyme and fecal fat studies ▪ Abnormal hydrogen breath test, d-xylose test ▪ Abnormal tests for inborn errors of metabolism
Anthropometric Measurements	▪ Weight loss of $\geq 5\%$ in one month, $\geq 10\%$ in six months ▪ Growth stunting or failure
Physical Exam Findings	▪ Abdominal distension ▪ Increased or decreased bowel sounds ▪ Evidence of vitamin and/or mineral deficiency, e.g., glossitis, cheilosis, mouth lesions
Food/Nutrition History	Reports or observations of: ▪ Avoidance or limitation of total intake or intake of specific foods/food groups due to GI symptoms, e.g., bloating, cramping, pain, diarrhea, steatorrhea (greasy, floating, foul-smelling stools) especially following ingestion of food
Client History	▪ Diarrhea, steatorrhea, abdominal pain ▪ Endoscopic or colonoscopic examination results, biopsy results ▪ Conditions associated with a diagnosis or treatment, e.g., malabsorption, maldigestion, cystic fibrosis, celiac disease, Crohn's disease, infection, radiation therapy, inborn errors of metabolism ▪ Surgical procedures, e.g., gastric bypass, bowel resection

CLINICAL

Edition: 2008

ALTERED NUTRITION-RELATED
LABORATORY VALUES (SPECIFY) (NC-2.2)

Definition
Changes due to body composition, medications, body system changes or genetics, or changes in ability to eliminate byproducts of digestive and metabolic processes.

Etiology (*Cause/Contributing Risk Factors*)
Factors gathered during the nutrition assessment process that contribute to the existence or the maintenance of pathophysiological, psychosocial, situational, developmental, cultural, and/or environmental problems:
- Kidney, liver, cardiac, endocrine, neurologic, and/or pulmonary dysfunction
- Other organ dysfunction that leads to biochemical changes

Signs/Symptoms (Defining Characteristics)
A typical cluster of subjective and objective signs and symptoms gathered during the nutrition assessment process that provide evidence that a problem exists; quantify the problem and describe its severity.

Nutrition Assessment Category	Potential Indicators of this Nutrition Diagnosis (one or more must be present)
Biochemical Data, Medical Tests and Procedures	▪ Increased AST, ALT, T. bili, serum ammonia (liver disorders) ▪ Abnormal BUN, Cr, K, phosphorus, glomerular filtration rate (GFR) (kidney disorders) ▪ Altered pO_2 and pCO_2 (pulmonary disorders) ▪ Abnormal serum lipids ▪ Abnormal plasma glucose and/or HgbA1c levels ▪ Inadequate blood glucose control ▪ Other findings of acute or chronic disorders that are abnormal and of nutritional origin or consequence
Anthropometric Measurements	▪ Rapid weight changes ▪ Other anthropometric measures that are altered
Physical Exam Findings	▪ Jaundice, edema, ascites, itching (liver disorders) ▪ Edema, shortness of breath (cardiac disorders) ▪ Blue nail beds, clubbing (pulmonary disorders)
Food/Nutrition History	Reports or observations of: ▪ Anorexia, nausea, vomiting ▪ Intake of foods high in or overall excess intake of protein, potassium, phosphorus, sodium, fluid ▪ Inadequate intake of micronutrients ▪ Food- and nutrition-related knowledge deficit, e.g., lack of information, incorrect information, or noncompliance with modified diet
Client History	▪ Conditions associated with a diagnosis or treatment, e.g., renal or liver disease, alcoholism, cardiopulmonary disorders, diabetes

Updated: 2008 Edition

FOOD–MEDICATION INTERACTION (NC-2.3)

Definition

Undesirable/harmful interaction(s) between food and over-the-counter (OTC) medications, prescribed medications, herbals, botanicals, and/or dietary supplements that diminishes, enhances, or alters effect of nutrients and/or medications.

Etiology (*Cause/Contributing Risk Factors*)

Factors gathered during the nutrition assessment process that contribute to the existence or the maintenance of pathophysiological, psychosocial, situational, developmental, cultural, and/or environmental problems:

- Combined ingestion or administration of medication and food that results in undesirable/harmful interaction

Signs/Symptoms (*Defining Characteristics*)

A typical cluster of subjective and objective signs and symptoms gathered during the nutrition assessment process that provide evidence that a problem exists; quantify the problem and describe its severity.

Nutrition Assessment Category	Potential Indicators of this Nutrition Diagnosis (one or more must be present)
Biochemical Data, Medical Tests and Procedures	▪ Alterations of biochemical tests based on medication affect and patient/client condition
Anthropometric Measurements	▪ Alterations of anthropometric measurements based on medication affect and patient/client conditions, e.g., weight gain and corticosteroids
Physical Exam Findings	
Food/Nutrition History	Reports or observations of: ▪ Intake that is problematic or inconsistent with OTC, prescribed drugs, herbals, botanicals, and dietary supplements, such as: • fish oils and prolonged bleeding • coumadin, vitamin K–rich foods • high-fat diet while on cholesterol-lowering medications • iron supplements, constipation and low-fiber diet ▪ Intake that does not support replacement or mitigation of OTC, prescribed drugs, herbals, botanicals, and dietary supplements affects such as potassium-wasting diuretics ▪ Changes in appetite or taste
Client History	▪ Multiple drugs (OTC, prescribed drugs, herbals, botanicals, and dietary supplements) that are known to have food–medication interactions ▪ Medications that require nutrient supplementation that can not be accomplished via food intake, e.g., isoniazid and vitamin B-6

UNDERWEIGHT (NC-3.1)

Definition
Low body weight compared to established reference standards or recommendations.

Etiology (*Cause/Contributing Risk Factors*)
Factors gathered during the nutrition assessment process that contribute to the existence or the maintenance of pathophysiological, psychosocial, situational, developmental, cultural, and/or environmental problems:

- Disordered eating pattern
- Excessive physical activity
- Harmful beliefs/attitudes about food, nutrition, and nutrition-related topics
- Inadequate energy intake
- Increased energy needs
- Limited access to food

Signs/Symptoms (*Defining Characteristics*)
A typical cluster of subjective and objective signs and symptoms gathered during the nutrition assessment process that provide evidence that a problem exists; quantify the problem and describe its severity.

Nutrition Assessment Category	Potential Indicators of this Nutrition Diagnosis (one or more must be present)
Biochemical Data, Medical Tests and Procedures	▪ Measured resting metabolic rate (RMR) measurement higher than expected and/or estimated RMR
Anthropometric Measurements	▪ Weight for age less than 5th percentile for infants younger than 12 months ▪ Decreased skinfold thickness and MAMC ▪ BMI < 18.5 (most adults) ▪ BMI for older adults (older than 65 years) < 23 ▪ BMI < 5th percentile (children, 2-19 years)
Physical Exam Findings	▪ Decreased muscle mass, muscle wasting (gluteal and temporal)
Food/Nutrition History	Reports or observations of: ▪ Inadequate intake of food compared to estimated or measured needs ▪ Limited supply of food in home ▪ Dieting, food faddism ▪ Hunger ▪ Refusal to eat ▪ Physical activity more than recommended amount ▪ Vitamin/mineral deficiency
Client History	▪ Malnutrition ▪ Illness or physical disability ▪ Mental illness, dementia, confusion ▪ Medications that affect appetite, e.g., stimulants for ADHD ▪ Athlete, dancer, gymnast

Updated: 2008 Edition

INVOLUNTARY WEIGHT LOSS (NC-3.2)

Definition
Decrease in body weight that is not planned or desired.

Etiology (*Cause/Contributing Risk Factors*)
Factors gathered during the nutrition assessment process that contribute to the existence or the maintenance of pathophysiological, psychosocial, situational, developmental, cultural, and/or environmental problems:

- Physiological causes, e.g., prolonged catabolic illness, trauma, malabsorption
- Lack of access to food, e.g., economic constraints, cultural or religious practices, restricting food given to elderly and/or children
- Prolonged hospitalization
- Psychological issues
- Lack of self-feeding ability

Signs/Symptoms (*Defining Characteristics*)
A typical cluster of subjective and objective signs and symptoms gathered during the nutrition assessment process that provide evidence that a problem exists; quantify the problem and describe its severity.

Nutrition Assessment Category	Potential Indicators of this Nutrition Diagnosis (one or more must be present)
Biochemical Data, Medical Tests and Procedures	
Anthropometric Measurements	▪ Weight loss of ≥ 5% within 30 days, ≥ 7.5% in 90 days, or ≥ 10% in 180 days
Physical Examination Findings	▪ Fever ▪ Decreased senses, i.e., smell, taste, vision ▪ Increased heart rate ▪ Increased respiratory rate ▪ Loss of subcutaneous fat and muscle stores
Food/Nutrition History	Reports or observations of: ▪ Normal or usual intake in face of illness ▪ Poor intake, change in eating habits, early satiety, skipped meals ▪ Change in way clothes fit
Client History	▪ Conditions associated with a diagnosis or treatment, e.g., AIDS/HIV, burns, chronic obstructive pulmonary disease, dysphagia, hip/long bone fracture, infection, surgery, trauma, hyperthyroidism (pre- or untreated), some types of cancer or metastatic disease (specify), substance abuse ▪ Changes in mental status or function (e.g., depression) ▪ Medications associated with weight loss, such as certain antidepressants or cancer chemotherapy

Updated: 2008 Edition

CLINICAL

OVERWEIGHT/OBESITY (NC-3.3)

Definition

Increased adiposity compared to established reference standards or recommendations, ranging from overweight to morbid obesity.

Etiology *(Cause/Contributing Risk Factors)*

Factors gathered during the nutrition assessment process that contribute to the existence or the maintenance of pathophysiological, psychosocial, situational, developmental, cultural, and/or environmental problems:

- Decreased energy needs
- Disordered eating pattern
- Excess energy intake
- Food- and nutrition-related knowledge deficit
- Not ready for diet/lifestyle change
- Physical inactivity
- Increased psychological/life stress

Signs/Symptoms *(Defining Characteristics)*

A typical cluster of subjective and objective signs and symptoms gathered during the nutrition assessment process that provide evidence that a problem exists; quantify the problem and describe its severity.

Nutrition Assessment Category	Potential Indicators of this Nutrition Diagnosis (one or more must be present)
Biochemical Data, Medical Tests and Procedures	▪ Measured resting metabolic rate (RMR) measurement less than expected and/or estimated RMR

Anthropometric Measurements	▪ BMI more than normative standard for age and gender
	  • Overweight 25-29.9
	  • Obesity-grade I 30-34.9
	  • Obesity-grade II 35-39.9
	  • Obesity-grade III 40+
	▪ Waist circumference more than normative standard for age and sex
	▪ Increased skinfold thickness
	▪ Weight for height more than normative standard for age and sex

Physical Exam Findings	▪ Increased body adiposity

OVERWEIGHT/OBESITY (NC-3.3)

Food/Nutrition History	Reports or observations of: • Overconsumption of high-fat and/or calorie-density food or beverage • Large portions of food (portion size more than twice than recommended) • Excessive energy intake • Infrequent, low-duration and/or low-intensity physical activity • Large amounts of sedentary activities, e.g., TV watching, reading, computer use in both leisure and work/school • Uncertainty regarding nutrition-related recommendations • Inability to apply nutrition-related recommendations • Inability to maintain weight or regain of weight • Unwillingness or disinterest in applying nutrition-related recommendations
Client History	• Conditions associated with a diagnosis or treatment, e.g., hypothyroidism, metabolic syndrome, eating disorder not otherwise specified, depression • Physical disability or limitation • History of familial obesity • History of childhood obesity • History of physical, sexual, or emotional abuse • Inability to lose a significant amount of excess weight through conventional weight loss intervention • Medications that impact RMR, e.g., midazolam, propranalol, glipizide

Updated: 2008 Edition

CLINICAL

INVOLUNTARY WEIGHT GAIN (NC-3.4)

Definition
Weight gain more than that which is desired or planned.

Etiology (*Cause/Contributing Risk Factors*)
Factors gathered during the nutrition assessment process that contribute to the existence or the maintenance of pathophysiological, psychosocial, situational, developmental, cultural, and/or environmental problems:

- Illness causing unexpected weight gain because of head trauma, immobility, paralysis or related condition
- Chronic use of medications known to cause weight gain, such as use of certain antidepressants, antipsychotics, corticosteroids, certain HIV medications
- Condition leading to excessive fluid weight gains

Signs/Symptoms (*Defining Characteristics*)
A typical cluster of subjective and objective signs and symptoms gathered during the nutrition assessment process that provide evidence that a problem exists; quantify the problem and describe its severity.

Nutrition Assessment Category	Potential Indicators of this Nutrition Diagnosis (one or more must be present)
Biochemical Data, Medical Tests and Procedures	▪ Decrease in serum albumin, hyponatremia, elevated fasting serum lipid levels, elevated fasting glucose levels, fluctuating hormone levels
Anthropometric Measurements	▪ Increased weight, any increase in weight more than planned or desired, such as 10% in 6 months ▪ Noticeable change in body fat distribution
Physical Examination Findings	▪ Fat accumulation, excessive subcutaneous fat stores ▪ Lipodystrophy associated with HIV diagnosis: increase in dorsocervial fat, breast enlargement, increased abdominal girth ▪ Edema ▪ Shortness of breath

INVOLUNTARY WEIGHT GAIN (NC-3.4)

Food/Nutrition History	Reports or observations of: • Intake consistent with estimated or measured energy needs • Changes in recent food intake level • Fluid administration more than requirements • Use of alcohol, narcotics • Extreme hunger with or without palpitations, tremor, and sweating • Physical inactivity or change in physical activity level
Client History	• Conditions associated with a diagnosis or treatment of asthma, psychiatric illnesses, rheumatic conditions, HIV/AIDS, Cushing's syndrome, obesity, Prader-Willi syndrome, hypothyroidism • Muscle weakness • Fatigue • Medications associated with increased appetite

Updated: 2008 Edition

FOOD- AND NUTRITION-RELATED
KNOWLEDGE DEFICIT (NB-1.1)

Definition

Incomplete or inaccurate knowledge about food, nutrition, or nutrition-related information and guidelines, e.g., nutrient requirements, consequences of food behaviors, life stage requirements, nutrition recommendations, diseases and conditions, physiological function, or products.

Etiology (*Cause/Contributing Risk Factors*)

Factors gathered during the nutrition assessment process that contribute to the existence or the maintenance of pathophysiological, psychosocial, situational, developmental, cultural, and/or environmental problems:

- Harmful beliefs/attitudes about food, nutrition, and nutrition-related topics
- Lack of prior exposure to information
- Language or cultural barrier impacting ability to learn information
- Learning disability, neurological or sensory impairment
- Prior exposure to incompatible information
- Prior exposure to incorrect information
- Unwilling or uninterested in learning information

Signs/Symptoms (*Defining Characteristics*)

A typical cluster of subjective and objective signs and symptoms gathered during the nutrition assessment process that provide evidence that a problem exists; quantify the problem and describe its severity.

Nutrition Assessment Category	Potential Indicators of this Nutrition Diagnosis (one or more must be present)
Biochemical Data, Medical Tests and Procedures	
Anthropometric Measurements	
Physical Exam Findings	
Food/Nutrition History	Reports or observations of: ■ Verbalizes inaccurate or incomplete information ■ Provides inaccurate or incomplete written response to questionnaire/written tool or is unable to read written tool ■ No prior knowledge of need for food- and nutrition-related recommendations ■ Demonstrates inability to apply food- and nutrition-related information, e.g., select food based on nutrition therapy or prepare infant feeding as instructed ■ Relates concerns about previous attempts to learn information ■ Verbalizes unwillingness or disinterest in learning information
Client History	■ Conditions associated with a diagnosis or treatment, e.g., mental illness ■ New medical diagnosis or change in existing diagnosis or condition

HARMFUL BELIEFS/ATTITUDES
ABOUT FOOD OR NUTRITION-RELATED TOPICS (NB-1.2)

Use with caution: Be sensitive to patient concerns.

Definition

Beliefs/attitudes or practices about food, nutrition, and nutrition-related topics that are incompatible with sound nutrition principles, nutrition care, or disease/condition (excluding disordered eating patterns and eating disorders).

Etiology *(Cause/Contributing Risk Factors)*

Factors gathered during the nutrition assessment process that contribute to the existence or the maintenance of pathophysiological, psychosocial, situational, developmental, cultural, and/or environmental problems:

- Disbelief in science-based food and nutrition information
- Exposure to incorrect food and nutrition information
- Eating behavior serves a purpose other than nourishment (e.g., pica)
- Desire for a cure for a chronic disease through the use of alternative therapy

Signs/Symptoms *(Defining Characteristics)*

A typical cluster of subjective and objective signs and symptoms gathered during the nutrition assessment process that provide evidence that a problem exists; quantify the problem and describe its severity.

Nutrition Assessment Category	Potential Indicators of this Nutrition Diagnosis (one or more must be present)
Biochemical Data, Medical Tests and Procedures	
Anthropometric Measurements	
Physical Exam Findings	
Food/Nutrition History	Reports or observations of: ▪ Food fetish, pica ▪ Food faddism ▪ Intake that reflects an imbalance of nutrients/food groups ▪ Avoidance of foods/food groups (e.g., sugar, wheat, cooked foods)
Client History	▪ Conditions associated with a diagnosis or treatment, e.g., obesity, diabetes, cancer, cardiovascular disease, mental illness

BEHAVIORAL

Edition: 2008

NOT READY FOR DIET/LIFESTYLE CHANGE (NB-1.3)

Definition
Lack of perceived value of nutrition-related behavior change compared to costs (consequences or effort required to make changes); conflict with personal value system; antecedent to behavior change.

Etiology (*Cause/Contributing Risk Factors*)
Factors gathered during the nutrition assessment process that contribute to the existence or the maintenance of pathophysiological, psychosocial, situational, developmental, cultural, and/or environmental problems:
- Harmful beliefs/attitudes about food, nutrition, and nutrition-related topics
- Cognitive deficits or inability to focus on dietary changes
- Lack of social support for implementing changes
- Denial of need to change
- Perception that time, interpersonal, or financial constraints prevent changes
- Unwilling or uninterested in learning information
- Lack of self-efficacy for making change or demoralization from previous failures at change

Signs/Symptoms (*Defining Characteristics*)
A typical cluster of subjective and objective signs and symptoms gathered during the nutrition assessment process that provide evidence that a problem exists; quantify the problem and describe its severity.

Nutrition Assessment Category	Potential Indicators of this Nutrition Diagnosis (one or more must be present)
Biochemical Data, Medical Tests and Procedures	
Anthropometric Measurements	
Physical Exam Findings	▪ Negative body language, e.g., frowning, lack of eye contact, defensive posture, lack of focus, fidgeting (Note: Body language varies by culture.)
Food/Nutrition History	Reports or observations of: ▪ Denial of need for food- and nutrition-related changes ▪ Inability to understand required changes ▪ Failure to keep appointments/schedule follow-up appointments or engage in counseling ▪ Previous failures to effectively change target behavior ▪ Defensiveness, hostility or resistance to change ▪ Lack of efficacy to make change or to overcome barriers to change
Client History	

Updated: 2008 Edition

SELF-MONITORING DEFICIT (NB-1.4)

Definition

Lack of data recording to track personal progress.

Etiology (*Cause/Contributing Risk Factors*)

Factors gathered during the nutrition assessment process that contribute to the existence or the maintenance of pathophysiological, psychosocial, situational, developmental, cultural, and/or environmental problems:

- Food- and nutrition-related knowledge deficit
- Lack of social support for implementing changes
- Lack of value for behavior change or competing values
- Perception that lack of resources (e.g., time, financial, or social support) prevent self-monitoring
- Cultural barrier impacting ability to track personal progress
- Learning disability, neurological, or sensory impairment
- Prior exposure to incompatible information
- Not ready for diet/lifestyle change
- Unwilling or uninterested in tracking progress
- Lack of focus and attention to detail, difficulty with time management and/or organization

Signs/Symptoms (*Defining Characteristics*)

A typical cluster of subjective and objective signs and symptoms gathered during the nutrition assessment process that provide evidence that a problem exists; quantify the problem and describe its severity.

Nutrition Assessment Category	Potential Indicators of this Nutrition Diagnosis (one or more must be present)
Biochemical Data, Medical Tests and Procedures	▪ Recorded data inconsistent with biochemical data, e.g., dietary intake is not consistent with biochemical data
Anthropometric Measurements	
Physical Exam Findings	

BEHAVIORAL

Edition: 2008

SELF-MONITORING DEFICIT CONT'D (NB-1.4)

Food/Nutrition History	Reports or observations of: • Incomplete self-monitoring records, e.g., glucose, food, fluid intake, weight, physical activity, ostomy output records • Food intake data inconsistent with weight status or growth pattern data • Embarrassment or anger regarding need for self-monitoring • Uncertainty of how to complete monitoring records • Uncertainty regarding changes that could/should be made in response to data in self-monitoring records • No self-management equipment, e.g., no blood glucose monitor, pedometer
Client History	• Diagnoses associated with self-monitoring, e.g., diabetes mellitus, obesity, new ostomy • New medical diagnosis or change in existing diagnosis or condition

DISORDERED EATING PATTERN (NB-1.5)

Definition

Beliefs, attitudes, thoughts, and behaviors related to food, eating, and weight management, including classic eating disorders as well as less severe, similar conditions that negatively impact health.

Etiology (*Cause/Contributing Risk Factors*)

Factors gathered during the nutrition assessment process that contribute to the existence or the maintenance of pathophysiological, psychosocial, situational, developmental, cultural, and/or environmental problems:

- Familial, societal, biological/genetic, and/or environmental related obsessive desire to be thin
- Weight regulation/preoccupation significantly influences self-esteem

Signs/Symptoms (*Defining Characteristics*)

A typical cluster of subjective and objective signs and symptoms gathered during the nutrition assessment process that provide evidence that a problem exists; quantify the problem and describe its severity.

Nutrition Assessment Category	Potential Indicators of this Nutrition Diagnosis (one or more must be present)
Biochemical Data, Medical Tests and Procedures	▪ Decreased cholesterol, abnormal lipid profiles, hypoglycemia, hypokalemia [anorexia nervosa (AN)] ▪ Hypokalemia and hypochloremic alkalosis [bulimia nervosa (BN)] ▪ Hyponatremia, hypothyroid, leukopenia, elevated BUN (AN) ▪ Urine positive for ketones (AN)
Anthropometric Measurements	▪ BMI < 17.5, arrested growth and development, failure to gain weight during period of expected growth, weight less than 85% of expected (AN) ▪ BMI > 29 [eating disorder not otherwise specified (EDNOS)] ▪ Significant weight fluctuation (BN)

BEHAVIORAL

Edition: 2008

DISORDERED EATING PATTERN CONT'D (NB-1.5)

Physical Exam Findings	• Severely depleted adipose and somatic protein stores (AN) • Lanugo hair formation on face and trunk, brittle listless hair, cyanosis of hands and feet, and dry skin (AN) • Normal or excess adipose and normal somatic protein stores (BN, EDNOS) • Damaged tooth enamel (BN) • Enlarged parotid glands (BN) • Peripheral edema (BN) • Skeletal muscle loss (AN) • Cardiac arrhythmias, bradycardia (AN, BN) • Hypotension, low body temperature • Inability to concentrate (AN) • Positive Russell's Sign (BN) callous on back of hand from self-induced vomiting • Bradycardia (heart rate < 60 beats/min), hypotension (systolic < 90 mm HG), and orthostatic hypotension (AN)
Food/Nutrition History	Reports or observations of: • Avoidance of food or calorie-containing beverages (AN, BN) • Fear of foods or dysfunctional thoughts regarding food or food experiences (AN, BN) • Denial of hunger (AN) • Food and weight preoccupation (AN, BN) • Knowledgeable about current diet fad (AN, BN, EDNOS) • Fasting (AN, BN) • Intake of larger quantity of food in a defined time period, a sense of lack of control over eating (BN, EDNOS) • Excessive physical activity (AN, BN, EDNOS) • Eating much more rapidly than normal, until feeling uncomfortably full, consuming large amounts of food when not feeling physically hungry; eating alone because of embarrassment, feeling very guilty after overeating (EDNOS) • Eats in private (AN, BN) • Irrational thoughts about food's affect on the body (AN, BN, EDNOS) • Pattern of chronic dieting • Excessive reliance on nutrition terming and preoccupation with nutrient content of foods • Inflexibility with food selection

DISORDERED EATING PATTERN (NB-1.5)

Client History	
	▪ Self-induced vomiting, diarrhea, bloating, constipation, and flatulence (BN); always cold (AN) ▪ Misuse of laxatives, enemas, diuretics, stimulants, and/or metabolic enhancers (AN,BN) ▪ Muscle weakness, fatigue, cardiac arrhythmias, dehydration, and electrolyte imbalance (AN, BN) ▪ Diagnosis, e.g., anorexia nervosa, bulimia nervosa, binge eating, eating disorder not otherwise specified, amenorrhea ▪ History of mood and anxiety disorders (e.g., depression, obsessive/compulsive disorder [OCD]), personality disorders, substance abuse disorders ▪ Family history of ED, depression, OCD, anxiety disorders (AN, BN) ▪ Irritability, depression (AN, BN) ▪ Anemia ▪ Avoidance of social events at which food is served

Edition: 2008

LIMITED ADHERENCE TO
NUTRITION-RELATED RECOMMENDATIONS (NB-1.6)

Definition
Lack of nutrition-related changes as per intervention agreed on by client or population.

Etiology (*Cause/Contributing Risk Factors*)
Factors gathered during the nutrition assessment process that contribute to the existence or the maintenance of pathophysiological, psychosocial, situational, developmental, cultural, and/or environmental problems:

- Lack of social support for implementing changes
- Lack of value for behavior change or competing values
- Perception that time or financial constraints prevent changes
- Previous lack of success in making health-related changes
- Poor understanding of how and why to make the changes
- Unwilling or uninterested in applying information

Signs/Symptoms (*Defining Characteristics*)
A typical cluster of subjective and objective signs and symptoms gathered during the nutrition assessment process that provide evidence that a problem exists; quantify the problem and describe its severity.

Nutrition Assessment Category	Potential Indicators of this Nutrition Diagnosis (one or more must be present)
Biochemical Data, Medical Tests and Procedures	▪ Expected laboratory outcomes are not achieved
Anthropometric Measurements	▪ Expected anthropometric outcomes are not achieved
Physical Exam Findings	▪ Negative body language, e.g., frowning, lack of eye contact, fidgeting (Note: body language varies by culture)
Food/Nutrition History	Reports or observations of: ▪ Expected food/nutrition-related outcomes are not achieved ▪ Inability to recall agreed on changes ▪ Failure to complete any agreed on homework ▪ Lack of compliance or inconsistent compliance with plan ▪ Failure to keep appointments or schedule follow-up appointments ▪ Lack of appreciation of the importance of making recommended nutrition-related changes ▪ Uncertainty as to how to consistently apply food/nutrition information
Client History	

BEHAVIORAL

UNDESIRABLE FOOD CHOICES (NB-1.7)

Definition

Food and/or beverage choices that are inconsistent with Dietary Reference Intakes (DRIs), US Dietary Guidelines, or My Pyramid, or with targets defined in the nutrition prescription or nutrition care process.

Etiology (*Cause/Contributing Risk Factors*)

Factors gathered during the nutrition assessment process that contribute to the existence or the maintenance of pathophysiological, psychosocial, situational, developmental, cultural, and/or environmental problems:

- Lack of prior exposure to or misunderstanding of information
- Language, religious, or cultural barrier impacting ability to apply information
- Learning disabilities, neurological or sensory impairment
- High level of fatigue or other side effect of medical, surgical or radiological therapy
- Inadequate access to recommended foods
- Perception that financial constraints prevent selection of food choices consistent with recommendations
- Food allergies and aversions impeding food choices consistent with guidelines
- Lacks motivation and or readiness to apply or support systems change
- Unwilling or uninterested in learning information
- Psychological limitations

Signs/Symptoms (*Defining Characteristics*)

A typical cluster of subjective and objective signs and symptoms gathered during the nutrition assessment process that provide evidence that a problem exists; quantify the problem and describe its severity.

Nutrition Assessment Category	Potential Indicators of this Nutrition Diagnosis (one or more must be present)
Biochemical Data, Medical Tests and Procedures	▪ Elevated lipid panel
Anthropometric Measurements	
Physical Exam Findings	▪ Findings consistent with vitamin/mineral deficiency or excess

Edition: 2008

UNDESIRABLE FOOD CHOICES CONT'D (NB-1.7)

Food/Nutrition History	Reports or observations of: • Intake inconsistent with DRIs, US Dietary Guidelines, MyPyramid, or other methods of measuring diet quality, such as, the Healthy Eating Index (e.g., omission of entire nutrient groups, disproportionate intake [e.g., juice for young children]) • Inaccurate or incomplete understanding of the guidelines • Inability to apply guideline information • Inability to select (e.g., access), or unwillingness, or disinterest in selecting, food consistent with the guidelines
Client History	• Conditions associated with a diagnosis or treatment, e.g., mental illness

Updated: 2008 Edition

BEHAVIORAL

PHYSICAL INACTIVITY (NB-2.1)

Definition

Low level of activity/sedentary behavior to the extent that it reduces energy expenditure and impacts health.

Etiology (*Cause/Contributing Risk Factors*)

Factors gathered during the nutrition assessment process that contribute to the existence or the maintenance of pathophysiological, psychosocial, situational, developmental, cultural, and/or environmental problems:

- Harmful beliefs/attitudes about physical activity
- Injury, lifestyle change, condition (e.g., advanced stages of cardiovascular disease, obesity, kidney disease), physical disability or limitation that reduces physical activity or activities of daily living
- Lack of knowledge about the health benefits of physical activity
- Lack of prior exposure regarding need for physical activity or how to incorporate exercise, e.g., physical disability, arthritis
- Lack of role models, e.g., for children
- Lack of social support and/or environmental space or equipment
- Lack of safe environment for physical activity
- Lack of value for behavior change or competing values
- Time constraints
- Financial constraints that may prevent sufficient level of activity (e.g., to address cost of equipment or shoes or club membership to gain access)

Signs/Symptoms (*Defining Characteristics*)

A typical cluster of subjective and objective signs and symptoms gathered during the nutrition assessment process that provide evidence that a problem exists; quantify the problem and describe its severity.

Nutrition Assessment Category	Potential Indicators of this Nutrition Diagnosis (one or more must be present)
Biochemical Data, Medical Tests and Procedures	
Anthropometric Measurements	▪ Obesity—BMI > 30 (adults), BMI > 95th percentile (pediatrics > 3 years)
Physical Exam Findings	▪ Excessive subcutaneous fat and low muscle mass

BEHAVIORAL

Edition: 2008

PHYSICAL INACTIVITY CONT'D (NB-2.1)

Food/Nutrition History	Reports or observations of: • Infrequent, low duration and/or low intensity physical activity • Large amounts of sedentary activities, e.g., TV watching, reading, computer use in both leisure and work/school • Low level of NEAT (non-exercise activity thermogenesis) expended by physical activities other than planned exercise, e.g., sitting, standing, walking, fidgeting
Client History	• Low cardiorespiratory fitness and/or low muscle strength • Medical diagnoses that may be associated with or result in decreased activity, e.g., arthritis, chronic fatigue syndrome, morbid obesity, knee surgery • Medications that cause somnolence and decreased cognition • Psychological diagnosis, e.g., depression, anxiety disorders

Updated: 2008 Edition

EXCESSIVE EXERCISE (NB-2.2)

Definition

An amount of exercise that exceeds that which is necessary to improve health and/or athletic performance.

Etiology (*Cause/Contributing Risk Factors*)

Factors gathered during the nutrition assessment process that contribute to the existence or the maintenance of pathophysiological, psychosocial, situational, developmental, cultural, and/or environmental problems:

- Disordered eating
- Irrational beliefs/attitudes about food, nutrition, and fitness
- "Addictive" behaviors/personality

Signs/Symptoms (*Defining Characteristics*)

A typical cluster of subjective and objective signs and symptoms gathered during the nutrition assessment process that provide evidence that a problem exists; quantify the problem and describe its severity.

Nutrition Assessment Category	Potential Indicators of this Nutrition Diagnosis (one or more must be present)
Biochemical Data, Medical Tests and Procedures	▪ Elevated liver enzymes, e.g., LDH, AST ▪ Altered micronutrient status, e.g., decreased serum ferritin, zinc, and insulin-like growth factor-binding protein ▪ Increased hematocrit ▪ Suppressed immune function ▪ Possibly elevated cortisol levels
Anthropometric Measurements	▪ Weight loss, arrested growth and development, failure to gain weight during period of expected growth (related usually to disordered eating)
Physical Exam Findings	▪ Depleted adipose and somatic protein stores (related usually to disordered eating) ▪ Frequent and/or prolonged injuries and/or illnesses ▪ Chronic muscle soreness
Food/Nutrition History	Reports or observations of: ▪ Continued/repeated high levels of exercise exceeding levels necessary to improve health and/or athletic performance ▪ Exercise daily without rest/rehabilitation days ▪ Exercise while injured/sick ▪ Forsaking family, job, social responsibilities to exercise ▪ Overtraining
Client History	▪ Conditions associated with a diagnosis or treatment, e.g., anorexia nervosa, bulimia nervosa, binge eating, eating disorder not otherwise specified, amenorrhea, stress fractures ▪ Chronic fatigue ▪ Evidence of addictive, obsessive, or compulsive tendencies

Updated: 2008 Edition

INABILITY OR LACK OF
DESIRE TO MANAGE SELF-CARE (NB-2.3)

Definition
Lack of capacity or unwillingness to implement methods to support healthful food-
and nutrition-related behavior.

Etiology (*Cause/Contributing Risk Factors*)
Factors gathered during the nutrition assessment process that contribute to the
existence or the maintenance of pathophysiological, psychosocial, situational,
developmental, cultural, and/or environmental problems:
- Food- and nutrition-related knowledge deficit
- Lack of caretaker or social support for implementing changes
- Lack of developmental readiness to perform self-management tasks, e.g.,
  pediatrics
- Lack of value for behavior change or competing values
- Perception that lack of resources (time, financial, support persons) prevent
  self-care
- Cultural beliefs and practices
- Learning disability, neurological or sensory impairment
- Prior exposure to incompatible information
- Not ready for diet/lifestyle change
- Unwilling or uninterested in learning/applying information
- No self-management tools or decision guides

Signs/Symptoms (*Defining Characteristics*)
A typical cluster of subjective and objective signs and symptoms gathered during the
nutrition assessment process that provide evidence that a problem exists; quantify
the problem and describe its severity.

Nutrition Assessment Category	Potential Indicators of this Nutrition Diagnosis (one or more must be present)
Biochemical Data, Medical Tests and Procedures	
Anthropometric Measurements	
Physical Exam Findings	
Food/Nutrition History	Reports or observations of: ▪ Inability to interpret data or self-management tools ▪ Embarrassment or anger regarding need for self-monitoring ▪ Uncertainty regarding changes could/should be made in response to data in self-monitoring records
Client History	▪ Diagnoses that are associated with self-management, e.g., diabetes mellitus, obesity, cardiovascular disease, renal or liver disease ▪ Conditions associated with a diagnosis or treatment, e.g., cognitive or emotional impairment ▪ New medical diagnosis or change in existing diagnosis or condition

IMPAIRED ABILITY TO PREPARE FOODS/MEALS (NB-2.4)

Definition
Cognitive or physical impairment that prevents preparation of foods/meals.

Etiology (*Cause/Contributing Risk Factors*)
Factors gathered during the nutrition assessment process that contribute to the existence or the maintenance of pathophysiological, psychosocial, situational, developmental, cultural, and/or environmental problems:

- Learning disability, neurological or sensory impairment
- Loss of mental or cognitive ability, e.g., dementia
- Physical disability
- High level of fatigue or other side effect of therapy

Signs/Symptoms (*Defining Characteristics*)
A typical cluster of subjective and objective signs and symptoms gathered during the nutrition assessment process that provide evidence that a problem exists; quantify the problem and describe its severity.

Nutrition Assessment Category	Potential Indicators of this Nutrition Diagnosis (one or more must be present)
Biochemical Data, Medical Tests and Procedures	
Anthropometric Measurements	
Physical Exam Findings	
Food/Nutrition History	Reports or observations of: ■ Decreased overall intake ■ Excessive consumption of convenience foods, pre-prepared meals, and foods prepared away from home resulting in an inability to adhere to nutrition prescription ■ Uncertainty regarding appropriate foods to prepare based on nutrition prescription ■ Inability to purchase and transport foods to one's home
Client History	■ Conditions associated with a diagnosis or treatment, e.g., cognitive impairment, cerebral palsy, paraplegia, vision problems, rigorous therapy regimen, recent surgery

BEHAVIORAL

Edition: 2008

POOR NUTRITION QUALITY OF LIFE (NQOL) (NB-2.5)

Definition
Diminished patient/client perception of quality of life in response to nutrition problems and recommendations.

Etiology (*Cause/Contributing Risk Factors*)
Factors gathered during the nutrition assessment process that contribute to the existence or the maintenance of pathophysiological, psychosocial, situational, developmental, cultural, and/or environmental problems:
- Food and nutrition knowledge–related deficit
- Not ready for diet/lifestyle change
- Negative impact of current or previous medical nutrition therapy (MNT)
- Food or activity behavior-related difficulty
- Poor self-efficacy
- Altered body image
- Food insecurity
- Lack of social support for implementing changes

Signs/Symptoms (*Defining Characteristics*)
A typical cluster of subjective and objective signs and symptoms gathered during the nutrition assessment process that provide evidence that a problem exists; quantify the problem and describe its severity.

Nutrition Assessment Category	Potential Indicators of this Nutrition Diagnosis (one or more must be present)
Biochemical Data, Medical Tests and Procedures	
Anthropometric Measurements	
Physical Exam Findings	

POOR NUTRITION QUALITY OF LIFE (NQOL) (NB-2.5)

Food/Nutrition History	Reports or observations of: ▪ Unfavorable NQOL rating ▪ Unfavorable ratings on measure of QOL, such as, SF36 (multi-purpose health survey form with 36 questions) or EORTC QLQ-C30 (quality of life tool developed for patient/clients with cancer) ▪ Food insecurity/unwillingness to use community services that are available ▪ Frustration or dissatisfaction with MNT recommendations ▪ Frustration over lack of control ▪ Inaccurate or incomplete information related to MNT recommendations ▪ Inability to change food- or activity-related behavior ▪ Concerns about previous attempts to learn information ▪ MNT recommendations effecting socialization ▪ Unwillingness or disinterest in learning information ▪ Lack of social and familial support ▪ Ethnic and cultural related issues
Client History	▪ New medical diagnosis or change in existing diagnosis or condition ▪ Recent other lifestyle or life changes, e.g., quit smoking, initiated exercise, work change, home relocation

Updated: 2008 Edition

BEHAVIORAL

SELF-FEEDING DIFFICULTY (NB-2.6)

Definition
Impaired actions to place food or beverages in mouth.

Etiology (*Cause/Contributing Risk Factors*)
Factors gathered during the nutrition assessment process that contribute to the existence or the maintenance of pathophysiological, psychosocial, situational, developmental, cultural, and/or environmental problems:

- Inability to grasp cups and utensils for self-feeding
- Inability to support and/or control head and neck
- Lack of coordination of hand to mouth
- Limited physical strength or range of motion
- Inability to bend elbow or wrist
- Inability to sit with hips square and back straight
- Limited access to foods and/or adaptive eating devices conducive for self-feeding
- Limited vision and/or impaired cognitive ability
- Reluctance or avoidance of self-feeding

Signs/Symptoms (*Defining Characteristics*)
A typical cluster of subjective and objective signs and symptoms gathered during the nutrition assessment process that provide evidence that a problem exists; quantify the problem and describe its severity.

Nutrition Assessment Category	Potential Indicators of this Nutrition Diagnosis (one or more must be present)
Biochemical Data, Medical Tests and Procedures	
Anthropometric Measurements	▪ Weight loss
Physical Exam Findings	▪ Dry mucous membranes, hoarse or wet voice, tongue extrusion

SELF-FEEDING DIFFICULTY (NB-2.6)

Food/Nutrition History	Reports or observations of:
	▪ Being provided with foods that may not be conducive to self-feeding, e.g., peas, broth-type soups
	▪ Poor lip closure, drooling
	▪ Dropping of cups, utensils
	▪ Emotional distress, anxiety, or frustration surrounding mealtimes
	▪ Failure to recognize foods
	▪ Forgets to eat
	▪ Inappropriate use of food
	▪ Refusal to eat or chew
	▪ Dropping of food from utensil (splashing and spilling of food) on repeated attempts to feed
	▪ Lack of strength or stamina to lift utensils and/or cup
	▪ Utensil biting
Client History	▪ Conditions associated with a diagnosis or treatment of, e.g., neurological disorders, Parkinson's, Alzheimer's, Tardive dyskinesia, multiple sclerosis, stroke, paralysis, developmental delay
	▪ Physical limitations, e.g., fractured arms, traction, contractures
	▪ Surgery requiring recumbent position
	▪ Dementia/organic brain syndrome
	▪ Dysphagia
	▪ Shortness of breath
	▪ Tremors

BEHAVIORAL

Updated: 2008 Edition

INTAKE OF UNSAFE FOOD (NB-3.1)

Definition

Intake of food and/or fluids intentionally or unintentionally contaminated with toxins, poisonous products, infectious agents, microbial agents, additives, allergens, and/or agents of bioterrorism.

Etiology (*Cause/Contributing Risk Factors*)

Factors gathered during the nutrition assessment process that contribute to the existence or the maintenance of pathophysiological, psychosocial, situational, developmental, cultural, and/or environmental problems:

- Lack of knowledge about potentially unsafe food
- Lack of knowledge about proper food/feeding, (infant and enteral formula, breast milk) storage and preparation
- Exposure to contaminated water or food, e.g., community outbreak of illness documented by surveillance and/or response agency
- Mental illness, confusion, or altered awareness
- Inadequate food storage equipment/facilities, e.g., refrigerator
- Inadequate safe food supply, e.g., inadequate markets with safe, uncontaminated food

Signs/Symptoms (*Defining Characteristics*)

A typical cluster of subjective and objective signs and symptoms gathered during the nutrition assessment process that provide evidence that a problem exists; quantify the problem and describe its severity.

Nutrition Assessment Category	Potential Indicators of this Nutrition Diagnosis (one or more must be present)
Biochemical Data, Medical Tests and Procedures	▪ Positive stool culture for infectious causes, such as listeria, salmonella, hepatitis A, E. coli, cyclospora ▪ Toxicology reports for drugs, medicinals, poisons in blood or food samples
Anthropometric Measurements	
Physical Examination Findings	▪ Evidence of dehydration, e.g., dry mucous membranes, damaged tissues

INTAKE OF UNSAFE FOOD (NB-3.1)

Food/Nutrition History	Reports or observations of intake of potential unsafe foods: ▪ Mercury content of fish, non-food items (pregnant and lactating women) ▪ Raw eggs, unpasteurized milk products, soft cheeses, undercooked meats (infants, children, immunocompromised persons, pregnant and lactating women, and elderly) ▪ Wild plants, berries, mushrooms ▪ Unsafe food/feeding storage and preparation practices (enteral and infant formula, breast milk)
Client History	▪ Conditions associated with a diagnosis or treatment, e.g., foodborne illness, such as, bacterial, viral, and parasitic infection, mental illness, dementia ▪ Poisoning by drugs, medicinals, and biological substances ▪ Poisoning from poisonous food stuffs and poisonous plants ▪ Diarrhea, cramping, bloating, fever, nausea, vomiting, vision problems, chills, dizziness, headache ▪ Cardiac, neurologic, respiratory changes

BEHAVIORAL

LIMITED ACCESS TO FOOD (NB-3.2)

Definition

Diminished ability to acquire a sufficient quantity and variety of healthful food based upon the U.S. Dietary Guidelines or MyPyramid. Limitation to food because of concerns about weight or aging.

Etiology (*Cause/Contributing Risk Factors*)

Factors gathered during the nutrition assessment process that contribute to the existence or the maintenance of pathophysiological, psychosocial, situational, developmental, cultural, and/or environmental problems:

- Caregiver intentionally or unintentionally not providing access to food, e.g., unmet needs for food or eating assistance, excess of poor nutritional quality food, abuse/neglect
- Community and geographical constraints for shopping and transportation
- Food and nutrition-related knowledge deficit
- Lack of financial resources or lack of access to financial resources to purchase a sufficient quantity or variety of culturally appropriate healthful foods
- Lack of food planning, purchasing, and preparation skills
- Limited, absent, or failure to participate in community supplemental food programs, e.g., food pantries, emergency kitchens, or shelters, with a sufficient variety of culturally appropriate healthful foods
- Failure to participate in federal food programs such as WIC, National School Breakfast/Lunch Program, food stamps
- Schools lacking nutrition/wellness policies or application of policies ensuring convenient, appetizing, competitively priced culturally appropriate healthful foods at meals, snacks, and school sponsored activities
- Physical or psychological limitations that diminish ability to shop, e.g., walking, sight, mental/emotional health

Signs/Symptoms (*Defining Characteristics*)

A typical cluster of subjective and objective signs and symptoms gathered during the nutrition assessment process that provide evidence that a problem exists; quantify the problem and describe its severity.

Nutrition Assessment Category	Potential Indicators of this Nutrition Diagnosis (one or more must be present)
Biochemical Data, Medical Tests and Procedures	▪ Indicators of macronutrient or vitamin/mineral status as indicated by physical findings, food/nutrition, and client history
Anthropometric Measurements	▪ Growth failure, based on National Center for Health Statistics (NCHS) growth standards ▪ Underweight (BMI < 18.5)

LIMITED ACCESS TO FOOD (NB-3.2)

Physical Exam Findings	▪ Findings consistent with vitamin/mineral deficiency
Food/Nutrition History	Reports or observations of: ▪ Food faddism or harmful beliefs and attitudes of parent or caregiver ▪ Belief that aging can be slowed by dietary limitations and extreme exercise ▪ Hunger ▪ Inadequate intake of food and/or specific nutrients ▪ Limited supply of food in home ▪ Limited variety of foods
Client History	▪ Malnutrition, vitamin/mineral deficiency ▪ Illness or physical disability ▪ Conditions associated with a diagnosis or treatment, e.g., mental illness, dementia ▪ Lack of suitable support systems

Updated: 2008 Edition

BEHAVIORAL

NCP Step 3. Nutrition Intervention

What is the purpose of a nutrition intervention? The purpose is to resolve or improve the identified nutrition problem by planning and implementing appropriate nutrition interventions that are tailored to the patient/client's* needs.

How does a dietetics practitioner determine a nutrition intervention? The selection of nutrition interventions is driven by the nutrition diagnosis and its etiology. Nutrition intervention strategies are purposefully selected to change nutritional intake, nutrition-related knowledge or behavior, environmental condition, or access to supportive care and services. Nutrition intervention goals provide the basis for monitoring progress and measuring outcomes.

How are the Nutrition Intervention strategies organized? In four categories:

Food and/or Nutrient Delivery—*An individualized approach for food/nutrient provision, including meals and snacks, enteral and parenteral feeding, and supplements*

Nutrition Education—*A formal process to instruct or train a patient/client in a skill or to impart knowledge to help patients/clients voluntarily manage or modify food choices and eating behavior to maintain or improve health*

Nutrition Counseling—*A supportive process, characterized by a collaborative counselor-patient relationship, to set priorities, establish goals and create individualized action plans that acknowledge and foster responsibility for self-care to treat an existing condition and promote health*

Coordination of Nutrition Care—*Consultation with, referral to, or coordination of nutrition care with other health care providers, institutions, or agencies that can assist in treating or managing nutrition-related problems*

What does Nutrition Intervention involve? Nutrition intervention entails two distinct and interrelated components—planning and implementing. Planning the nutrition intervention involves: a) prioritizing nutrition diagnoses, b) consulting ADA's *MNT Evidence-Based Guides for Practice* and other practice guides, c) determining patient-focused expected outcomes for each nutrition diagnosis, d) conferring with patient/client/caregivers, e) defining a nutrition intervention plan and strategies, f) defining time and frequency of care, and g) identifying resources needed. Implementation is the action phase and involves: a) communication of the nutrition care plan, b) carrying out the plan.

*Patient/client refers to individuals, groups, family members, and/or caregivers.

Are dietetics practitioners limited to the Nutrition Interventions listed in this reference? Nutrition intervention terminology includes commonly used strategies and emphasizes the application of evidence-based strategies matched to appropriate circumstances. Evaluation of the nutrition intervention terminology is ongoing and will guide future modifications. Dietetics practitioners can propose additions or revisions using the Procedure for Nutrition Controlled Vocabulary/ Terminology Maintenance/Review available from ADA.

Detailed information about this step can be found in the International Dietetics and Nutrition Terminology (IDNT) Reference Manual: Standardized Language for the Nutrition Care Process, First Edition, American Dietetic Association.

INTERVENTION

MEALS AND SNACKS (ND-1)

Definition

Meals are defined as regular eating events that include a variety of foods consisting of grains and/or starches, meat and/or meat alternatives, fruits and vegetables, and milk or milk products. A snack is defined as food served between regular meals.

Details of Intervention

A typical intervention might be further described with the following details:

- Recommend, implement, or order an appropriate distribution of type or quantity of food and nutrients within meals or at specified times
- Identify specific food/beverage(s) or groups for meals and snacks

See reference manual for list of nutrition diagnoses, etiologies and signs and symptoms that often are associated with this intervention.

Other considerations (*e.g., patient/client negotiation, patient/client needs and desires, and readiness to change*)

- Compliance skills and abilities
- Economic concerns with purchasing special food items
- Willingness/ability to change behavior to comply with diet
- Availability/access to a qualified practitioner for follow-up and monitoring

FOOD/
NUTRIENT

ENTERAL AND PARENTERAL NUTRITION (ND-2)

Definition

Enteral nutrition is defined as nutrition provided through the gastrointestinal (GI) tract via tube, catheter, or stoma that delivers nutrients distal to the oral cavity. Parenteral nutrition is defined as the administration of nutrients intravenously, centrally (delivered into a large-diameter vein, usually the superior vena cava adjacent to the right atrium) or peripherally (delivered into a peripheral vein, usually of the hand or forearm).

Details of Intervention

A typical intervention might be further described with the following details:

- Recommend, implement, or order changes in the rate, composition, schedule, and/or duration of feeding
- Recommend, implement, or order the initiation, route, and discontinuation of enteral nutrition
- Insert the feeding tube, provide tube site care; administer feedings
- Change dressings and provide line care
- Review changes in the intervention with the patient/client(s) and/or caregivers

See reference manual for list of nutrition diagnoses, etiologies and signs and symptoms that often are associated with this intervention.

Other considerations (*e.g., patient/client negotiation, patient/client needs and desires, and readiness to change*)

- End-of-life issues, ethical considerations, patient/client rights and family/caregiver issues.
- Other nutrient intake (oral, parenteral, or enteral nutrition)
- Enteral formulary composition and product availability
- Availability/access to a qualified practitioner for follow-up and monitoring
- Economic constraints that limit availability of food/enteral/parenteral products

FOOD/
NUTRIENT

Edition: 2008

MEDICAL FOOD SUPPLEMENTS (ND-3.1)

Definition

Commercial or prepared foods or beverages intended to supplement energy, protein, carbohydrate, fiber, and/or fat intake that may also contribute to vitamin and mineral intake.

Details of Intervention

A typical intervention might be further described with the following details:

- Recommend, implement, or order changes in an individualized feeding plan including the initiation, composition, type, frequency, timing, and discontinuation of oral supplements
- Describe the purpose of the supplement (e.g., to supplement energy, protein, carbohydrate, fiber, and/or fat intake)

See reference manual for list of nutrition diagnoses, etiologies and signs and symptoms that often are associated with this intervention.

Other considerations (*e.g., patient/client negotiation, patient/client needs and desires, and readiness to change*)

- Appetite sufficient to take medical food supplements
- System constraints that prevent meeting the client's preferences for specific flavors, textures, foods and the timing of feedings
- Availability of feeding assistance
- Economic concerns and product/food availability

FOOD/
NUTRIENT

VITAMIN OR MINERAL SUPPLEMENTS (ND-3.2)

Definition
A product that is intended to supplement vitamin or mineral intake.

Details of Intervention
A typical intervention might be further described with the following details:
- Recommend, implement, or order initiation, change in administration schedule and dose/form/route, or discontinuation of a vitamin and/or mineral supplement

See reference manual for list of nutrition diagnoses, etiologies and signs and symptoms that often are associated with this intervention.

Other considerations (*e.g., patient/client negotiation, patient/client needs and desires, and readiness to change*)
- Emerging scientific evidence to support the use of vitamin and mineral supplements in specific populations
- Availability of a qualified practitioner with additional education/training in the use of vitamin and mineral supplements in practice
- Economic considerations and product availability

FOOD/ NUTRIENT

Edition: 2008

BIOACTIVE SUBSTANCE SUPPLEMENT (ND-3.3)

Definition

A product that is intended to supplement bioactive substances (e.g., plant stanol and sterol esters, psyllium).

Details of Intervention

A typical intervention might be further described with the following details:

- Recommend, implement, or order initiation, changed in administration schedule or dose/form/route, or discontinuation of a bioactive substances (e.g., soluble fiber, soy protein, fish oils, plant sterol and stanol esters)

See reference manual for list of nutrition diagnoses, etiologies and signs and symptoms that often are associated with this intervention.

Other considerations (*e.g., patient/client negotiation, patient/client needs and desires, and readiness to change*)

- Emerging scientific evidence to support the use of bioactive supplements in specific populations
- Availability of a qualified practitioner with additional education/training in the use of bioactive supplements in practice

FOOD/
NUTRIENT

FEEDING ASSISTANCE (ND-4)

Definition

Accommodation or assistance in eating designed to restore the patient /client's ability to eat independently, support adequate nutrient intake, and reduce the incidence of unplanned weight loss and dehydration.

Details of Intervention

A typical intervention might be further described with the following details:

- Recommend, implement, or order adaptive equipment, feeding position, feeding cues, meal set-up, or mouth care to facilitate eating
- Recommend, design, or implement a restorative dining program
- Recommend, design, or implement a feeding assistance training program
- Recommends, designs, or implements menu selections that foster, promote, and maintain independent eating

See reference manual for list of nutrition diagnoses, etiologies and signs and symptoms that often are associated with this intervention.

Other considerations (*e.g., patient/client negotiation, patient/client needs and desires, and readiness to change*)

- Acceptance of feeding assistance/feeding devices
- Poor environment to foster adequate intake
- Lack of individual to provide assistance at meal time
- Lack of training in methods of feeding assistance
- Lack of available physical therapy, occupational therapy, or speech therapy evaluations
- Ability to understand the reasoning behind the recommendations and then want to make personal changes

FOOD/ NUTRIENT

Edition: 2008

FEEDING ENVIRONMENT (ND-5)

Definition

Adjustment of the physical environment, temperature, convenience, and attractiveness of the location where food is served that impacts food consumption.

Details of Intervention

A typical intervention might be further described with the following details:

- Recommend, implement, or order changes in table service/colors/set up/height, room temperature and lighting, meal schedule, menu choice, appetite enhancers, proper positioning, and minimize distractions and odors
- Recommend, implement, or order seating arrangements considering groupings that inspire social interactions

See reference manual for list of nutrition diagnoses, etiologies and signs and symptoms that often are associated with this intervention

Other considerations (*e.g., patient/client negotiation, patient/client needs and desires, and readiness to change*)

- Resources available to improve/modify the feeding environment

NUTRITION-RELATED MEDICATION MANAGEMENT (ND-6)

Definition
Modification of a drug or herbal to optimize patient/client nutritional or health status.

Details of Intervention
A typical intervention might be further described with the following details:
* Recommend, implement, order initiation, changes in dose/form/route, change in administration schedule, or discontinuance of medications or herbals including insulin, appetite stimulants, digestive enzymes, or probiotics

See reference manual for list of nutrition diagnoses, etiologies and signs and symptoms that often are associated with this intervention.

Other considerations (*e.g., patient/client negotiation, patient/client needs and desires, and readiness to change*)
* Availability/access to a clinical pharmacist
* Availability of a qualified practitioner with appropriate pharmacology training and/or education

FOOD/
NUTRIENT

Edition: 2008

INITIAL/BRIEF NUTRITION EDUCATION (E-1)

Definition

Instruction or training intended to build or reinforce basic nutrition-related knowledge, or to provide essential nutrition-related information until patient/client returns.

Details of Intervention

A typical intervention might be further described related the following details:

- Discuss the purpose of the nutrition education intervention
- Communicate relationship between nutrition and specific disease/health issue
- Begin instruction of nutrition issue of most concern to patient/client's health and well-being
- Provide basic nutrition-related educational information until client is able to return for comprehensive education

See reference manual for list of nutrition diagnoses, etiologies and signs and symptoms that often are associated with this intervention.

Other considerations (*e.g., patient/client negotiation, patient/client needs and desires, and readiness to change*)

- Met with several providers in one day and is unable or unwilling to receive more nutrition education at this time
- Profile reflects complicated situation warranting additional education/ instruction
- Being discharged from the hospital
- Caregiver unavailable at time of nutrition education
- Baseline knowledge
- Learning style
- Other education and learning needs, e.g., new medication or other treatment administration

EDUCATION

COMPREHENSIVE NUTRITION EDUCATION (E-2)

Definition

Instruction or training intended to lead to in-depth nutrition-related knowledge and/ or skills in given topics.

Details of Intervention

A typical intervention might be further described with the following details:

- Provide information related to purpose of the nutrition prescription
- Initiate thorough instruction of relationship between nutrition and disease/ health
- Explain detailed or multiple nutrition prescription modifications recommended given patient/client situation
- Introduce more advanced nutrition topics related to patient/condition (e.g., saturated and *trans* fatty acid intake vs. total fat intake, menu planning, food purchasing)
- Support skill development (e.g., glucometer use, home tube feeding and feeding pump training, cooking skills/preparation)
- Commence training on interpreting medical or other results to modify nutrition prescription (e.g., distribution of carbohydrates throughout the day based on blood glucose monitoring results)

See reference manual for list of nutrition diagnoses, etiologies and signs and symptoms that often are associated with this intervention.

Other considerations (*e.g., patient/client negotiation, patient/client needs and desires, and readiness to change*)

- Profile reflects complicated situation warranting additional education/ instruction
- Increased capacity and willingness to learn information
- Quality of life may be enhanced with in-depth nutrition education and understanding
- Baseline knowledge
- Lifestyle factors
- Education approaches that enhance knowledge/skill transfer

EDUCATION

Edition: 2008

THEORETICAL BASIS/APPROACH (C-1)

Definition

The theories or models used to design and implement an intervention. Theories and theoretical models consist of principles, constructs and variables, which offer systematic explanations of the human behavior change process. Behavior change theories and models provide a research-based rationale for designing and tailoring nutrition interventions to achieve the desired effect. A theoretical framework for curriculum and treatment protocols, it guides determination of: 1) what information patients/clients need at different points in the behavior change process, 2) what tools and strategies may be best applied to facilitate behavior change, and 3) outcome measures to assess effectiveness in interventions or components of interventions.

Application Guidance

One or more of the following theories or theoretical models may influence a practitioner's counseling style or approach. Practitioners are asked to identify those theories (C-1) that most influence the intervention being documented. An intervention might also incorporate tools and strategies derived from a variety of behavior change theories and models. The practitioner is also asked to indicate which strategies (C-2) they used in a particular intervention session.

Details of Intervention

A typical intervention might be further described with the following details:

The following theories and models have proven valuable in providing a theoretical framework for evidence-based individual and interpersonal level nutrition interventions. Other theories may be useful for community level interventions (e.g., Community Organization, Diffusion of Innovations, Communication Theory).

- Cognitive-Behavioral Theory
- Health Belief Model
- Social Learning Theory
- Transtheoretical Model/Stages of Change

Additional information regarding each of the above theories and models can be found within this reference sheet.

See reference manual for list of nutrition diagnoses, etiologies and signs and symptoms that often are associated with this intervention.

Other considerations (*e.g., patient/client negotiation, patient/client needs and desires, and readiness to change*)

- Lifestyle factors
- Language barrier
- Educational level
- Culture
- Socioeconomic status

COUNSELING

THEORETICAL BASIS/APPROACH (C-1)

Cognitive-Behavioral Theory

Description

Cognitive-behavioral theory (CBT) is based on the assumption that all behavior is learned and is directly related to internal factors (e.g., thoughts and thinking patterns) and external factors (e.g., environmental stimulus and reinforcement) that are related to the problem behaviors. Application involves use of both cognitive and behavioral change strategies to effect behavior change.

Implication for Counseling Interventions

CBT, derived from an educational model, is based upon the assumption that most emotional and behavioral reactions are learned and can be unlearned. The goal of CBT is to facilitate client identification of cognitions and behaviors that lead to inappropriate eating or exercise habits and replace these with more rational thoughts and actions.

The process is:

• Goal directed
• Process oriented
• Facilitated through a variety of problem solving tools

Behavioral and cognitive techniques to modify eating and exercise habits are taught for continuous application by the patient/client. Practitioners implement Cognitive-Behavioral Theory by partnering with clients to study their current environment to:

• Identify determinants or antecedents to behavior that contribute to inappropriate eating/exercise
• Identify resultant inappropriate behavior (e.g., overeating, vomiting)
• Analyze consequences of this behavior (cognitions, positive and negative reinforcers and punishments, e.g., decreased anxiety, feeling over full, losing or gaining weight)
• Make specific goals to modify the environment/cognitions to reduce target behaviors

Cognitive and behavioral strategies used to promote change in diet and physical activity may include:

• Goal setting
• Self-monitoring
• Problem solving
• Social support
• Stress management
• Stimulus control
• Cognitive restructuring
• Relapse prevention
• Rewards/contingency management

COUNSELING

Edition: 2008

THEORETICAL BASIS/APPROACH (C-1)

Health Belief Model

Description

The Health Belief Model is a psychological model, which focuses on an individual's attitudes and beliefs to attempt to explain and predict health behaviors. The HBM is based on the assumption that an individual will be motivated to take health-related action if that person 1) feels that a negative health condition (e.g., diabetes) can be avoided or managed, 2) has a positive expectation that by taking a recommended action, he/she will avoid negative health consequences (e.g., good blood glucose control will preserve eye sight), and believes he/she can successfully perform a recommended health action (e.g., I can use carbohydrate counting and control my diet).

Implication for Counseling Interventions

The Health Belief Model is particularly helpful to practitioners planning interventions targeted to individuals with clinical nutrition-related risk factors, such as diabetes, high blood cholesterol and/or hypertension. The six major constructs of the model have been found to be important in impacting an individual's motivation to take health-related action. The following page provides definitions and application guidance for the key constructs of the theory. Motivational interviewing strategies may be appropriate to address perceived susceptibility, severity, benefits and barriers. Behavioral strategies are most appropriate once the patient/client begins to take action to modify his/her diet.

These six constructs are useful components in designing behavior change programs. It is important for the practitioner to understand the patient's perception of the health threat and potential benefits of treatment. According to the HBM, an asymptomatic diabetic may not be compliant with his/her treatment regiment if he/she does not:

- believe he or she has diabetes (susceptibility)
- believe diabetes will seriously impact his/her life (perceived seriousness)
- believe following the diabetic diet will decrease the negative effects of diabetes (perceived benefits)
- believe the effort to follow the diet is worth the benefit to be gained (perceived barriers)
- have stimulus to initiate action (cue to action)
- have confidence in their ability to achieve success (self-efficacy)

COUNSELING

THEORETICAL BASIS/APPROACH (C-1)
Health Belief Model

Constructs

Perceived susceptibility
Client's belief or opinion of the personal threat a health condition represents for them; client opinion regarding whether they have the condition (e.g., diabetes or hypertension) or their chance of getting the disease or condition

Strategies
- Educate on disease/condition risk factors
- Tailor information to the client
- Ask client if they think they are at risk or have the disease/condition
- Guided discussions
- Motivational interviewing (express empathy, open-ended questions, reflective listening, affirming, summarizing, and eliciting self-motivation statements)

Perceived severity
Client's belief about the impact a particular health threat will have on them and their lifestyle

Strategies
- Educate on consequences of the disease/condition; show graphs, statistics
- Elicit client response
- Discuss potential impact on client's lifestyle
- Motivational interviewing

Perceived benefits and barriers
Client's belief regarding benefits they will derive from taking nutrition-related action; perceived benefits versus barriers—client's perception of whether benefits will outweigh the sacrifices and efforts involved in behavior change

Strategies
- Clearly define benefits of nutrition therapy
- Role models, testimonials
- Explore ambivalence and barriers
- Imagine the future
- Explore successes
- Summarize and affirm the positive

Cues to action
Internal or external triggers that motivate or stimulate action

Strategies
- How-to education
- Incentive programs
- Link current symptoms to disease/condition
- Discuss media information
- Reminder phone calls/mailings
- Social support

Self-efficacy
Client confidence in their ability to successfully accomplish the necessary action

Strategies
- Skill training/demonstration
- Introduce alternatives and choices
- Behavior contracting; small, incremental goals
- Coaching, verbal reinforcement

COUNSELING

THEORETICAL BASIS/APPROACH (C-1)

Social Learning Theory

Description

Social learning theory, also known as Social Cognitive Theory, provides a framework for understanding, predicting, and changing behavior. The theory identifies a dynamic, reciprocal relationship between environment, the person, and behavior. The person can be both an agent for change and a responder to change. It emphasizes the importance of observing and modeling behaviors, attitudes and emotional reactions of others. Determinants of behavior include goals, outcome expectations and self-efficacy. Reinforcements increase or decrease the likelihood that the behavior will be repeated.[1]

Implication for Counseling Interventions

Social Learning Theory is rich in concepts applicable to nutrition counseling. The following page provides definitions and application guidance for the key concepts of the theory.

THEORETICAL BASIS/APPROACH (C-1)

Social Learning Theory

Concepts

Reciprocal Determinism

A person's ability to change a behavior is influenced by characteristics within the person (e.g., beliefs), the environment, and the behavior itself (e.g., difficulty doing the behavior). All three interact to influence if the behavior change will happen.

Strategies

Consider multiple behavior change strategies targeting motivation, action, the individual and the environment:

- Motivational interviewing
- Social support
- Stimulus control
- Demonstration
- Skill development training/coaching

Behavioral Capability

The knowledge and skills that are needed for a person to change behavior

Strategies

- Comprehensive education
- Demonstration
- Skill development training/coaching

Expectations

For a person to do a behavior, they must believe that the behavior will result in outcomes important to them

Strategies

- Motivational interviewing
- Model positive outcomes of diet/exercise

Self-Efficacy

Confidence in ability to take action and persist in action

Strategies

- Break task down to component parts
- Demonstration/modeling
- Skill development training/coaching
- Reinforcement
- Small, incremental goals/behavioral contracting

Observational Learning

When a person learns how to do a behavior by watching credible others do the same behavior

Strategies

- Demonstrations
- Role modeling
- Group problem-solving sessions

Reinforcement

Response to a behavior that will either increase or decrease the likelihood that the behavior will be repeated

Strategies

- Affirm accomplishments
- Encourage self reward/self-reinforcement
- Incentives for process components of change (e.g., keeping a food diary)

THEORETICAL BASIS/APPROACH (C-1)
Transtheoretical Model/Stages of Change

Definition

A theoretical model of intentional health behavior change that describes a sequence of cognitive (attitudes and intentions) and behavioral steps people take in successful behavior change. The model, developed by Prochaska and DiClemente, is composed of a core concept known as Stages of Change, a series of independent variables, the Processes of Change, and outcome measures including decision balance and self-efficacy. The model has been used to guide development of effective interventions for a variety of health behaviors.

Implication for Counseling Interventions

One of the defining characteristics of this model is that it describes behavior change not as a discrete event (e.g., today I am going to stop overeating), but as something that occurs in stages, over time. The five stages reflect an individual's attitudes, intentions and behavior related to change of a specific behavior and include the following:

- Precontemplation—no recognition of need for change; no intention to take action within the next 6 months
- Contemplation—recognition of need to change; intends to take action within the next 6 months
- Preparation—intends to take action in the next 30 days and has taken some behavioral steps in that direction
- Action—has made changes in target behavior for less than 6 months
- Maintenance—has changed target behavior for more than 6 months

Determination of a patient/client stage of change is relatively simple, involving a few questions regarding intentions and current diet. One of the appealing aspects of the theory is that the Process of Change construct describes cognitive and behavioral activities or strategies, which may be applied at various stages to move a person forward through the stages of change. This movement is not always linear, and patients can cycle in and out of various stages. The model has been used to effectively tailor interventions to the needs of clients at various stages. Knowing a patient/client's stage of change can help a practitioner determine:

- Whether intervention now is appropriate
- The type and content of intervention to use (motivational versus action oriented)
- Appropriate and timely questions about past efforts, pros and cons of change, obstacles, challenges and potential strategies
- The amount of time to spend with the patient

The following table provides guidance for applying stages and processes of change to the adoption of healthy diets.

THEORETICAL BASIS/APPROACH (C-1)

General guidelines for applying stages and processes of change to adoption of healthful diets

State of readiness (Key strategies for moving to next stage)	Treatment do's and don'ts at this stage
Precontemplation (Increased information and awareness, emotional acceptance)	• Provide personalized information. • Allow client to express emotions about his or her disease or about the need to make dietary changes. • Do no assume the client has knowledge or expect that providing information will automatically lead to behavior change. • Do not ignore client's emotional adjustment to the need for dietary change, which could override ability to process relevant information.
Contemplation (Increased confidence in one's ability to adopt recommended behaviors)	• Discuss and resolve barriers to dietary change. • Encourage support networks. • Give positive feedback about a client's abilities. • Help to clarify ambivalence about adopting behavior and emphasize expected benefits. • Do not ignore the potential impact of family members, and others, on client's ability to comply. • Do not be alarmed by or critical of a client's ambivalence.
Preparation (Resolution of ambivalence, firm commitment, and specific action plan)	• Encourage client to set specific, achievable goals (e.g., use 1% milk instead of whole milk). • Reinforce small changes that client may have already achieved. • Do not recommend general behavior changes (e.g., "Eat less fat"). • Do not refer to small changes as "not good enough."
Action (Behavioral skill training and social support)	• Refer to education program for self-management skills. • Provide self-help materials. • Do not refer clients to information-only classes.
Maintenance (Problem-solving skills and social and environmental support)	• Encourage client to anticipate and plan for potential difficulties (e.g., maintaining dietary changes on vacation). • Collect information about local resources (e.g., support groups, shopping guides). • Encourage client to "recycle" if he or she has a lapse or relapse. • Recommend more challenging dietary changes if client is motivated. • Do not assume that initial action means permanent change. • Do not be discouraged or judgmental about a lapse or relapse.

Source: Adapted from Kristal AR, Glanz K, Curry S, Patterson RE. How can stages of change be best used in dietary interventions? *J Am Diet Assoc*. 1999;99:683.

Prochaska recommends the following strategies, which target motivation, be used in the early stages of change: consciousness raising, dramatic relief (e.g., emotional arousal via role playing or personal testimonials), environmental reevaluation (e.g., empathy training and family interactions), social liberation (e.g., advocacy, empowerment) and self-reevaluation (e.g., value clarification, healthy role models and imagery). These strategies are very consistent with motivational interviewing techniques. In the later stages of change, behavioral strategies are most appropriate.

STRATEGIES (C-2)

Definition

An evidence-based method or plan of action designed to achieve a particular goal. Application of behavior change theories in nutrition practice has provided practitioners with a collection of evidence-based strategies to promote behavior change. Some strategies target change in motivation and intention to change, and others target behavior change. Practitioners selectively apply strategies based upon patient/client goals and objectives, and their personal counseling philosophy and skill.

Application Guidance

An intervention typically incorporate tools and strategies derived from a variety of behavior change theories and models. The practitioner is asked to indicate which strategies (C-2) he/she used in a particular intervention session along with the theories (C-1), which most influence the intervention being documented.

Details of Intervention

A typical intervention might be further described with the following details:

The following strategies have proven valuable in providing effecting nutrition-related behavior change.

- Motivational interviewing
- Goal setting
- Self-monitoring
- Problem solving
- Social support
- Stress management
- Stimulus control
- Cognitive restructuring
- Relapse prevention
- Rewards/contingency management

Additional information regarding each of the above strategies can be found within this reference sheet.

See reference manual for list of nutrition diagnoses, etiologies and signs and symptoms that often are associated with this intervention

Other considerations (*e.g., patient/client negotiation, patient/client needs and desires, and readiness to change*)

- Lifestyle factors
- Language barrier
- Educational level
- Culture
- Socioeconomic status

STRATEGIES (C-2)

Strategy descriptions and application guidance

Motivational interviewing

A directive, client-centered counseling style for eliciting behavior change by helping clients to explore and resolve ambivalence.[1] The approach involves selective response to client speech in a way that helps the client resolve ambivalence and move toward change. The four guiding principles that underlie this counseling approach include:

- Express empathy
- Develop discrepancy
- Roll with resistance
- Support self-efficacy

The following specific practitioner behaviors are characteristic of the MI style:[2]

- Expressing acceptance and affirmation
- Eliciting and selectively reinforcing the client's own self motivational statements, expressions of problem recognition, concern, desire, intention to change, and ability to change
- Monitoring the client's degree of readiness to change, and ensuring that jumping ahead of the client does not generate resistance
- Affirming the client's freedom of choice and self-direction

The source of motivation is presumed to reside within the client and the counselor encourages the client to explore ambivalence, motivation and possibilities to change, so it is the client who chooses what to change, determines the change plan and strategy.

MI is an evidence-based counseling strategy which builds on Carl Roger's client-centered counseling model, Prochaska and DiClemente's transtheoretical model of change, Milton Rokeach's human values theory and Daryl Bern's theory of self-perception.

Implementation Tips

Tone of counseling:

- Partnership
- Nonjudgmental
- Empathetic/supportive/encouraging
- Nonconfrontational
- Quiet and eliciting

The client does most of the talking and the counselor guides the client to explore and resolve ambivalence by:

- Asking open ended questions
- Listening reflectively
- Summarizing
- Affirming
- Eliciting self-motivational statements
- Shared agenda setting/decision making
- Allowing clients to interpret information
- Rolling with resistance, rather than confronting
- Building discrepancy
- Eliciting "change talk"
- Negotiating a change plan

COUNSELING

STRATEGIES (C-2)

*Motivational interviewing is best applied in situations when a patient is not ready, is unwilling or ambivalent about changing their diet or lifestyle.

MI integrates well with the readiness to change model to move individuals from the early stages to the action stage of change.

MI is a major paradigm change from the problem solving oriented counseling frequently employed by practitioners.

MI is not a set of techniques that can be learned quickly, but a style or approach to counseling.

Goal setting
A collaborative activity between the client and the practitioner in which the client decides from all potential activity recommendations what changes he/she will expend effort to implement.

Implementation Tips
- Appropriate for patients ready to make dietary changes
- Coach on goal setting skills
- Document and track progress toward short-term and long-term goals
- Probe client about pros and cons of proposed goals
- Assist client in gaining the knowledge and skills necessary to succeed
- Encourage strategies to build confidence (discuss realistic steps and start with easily achievable goals)
- Aid clients in building a supportive environment
- Celebrate successes

Self-monitoring
A technique that involves keeping a detailed record of behaviors that influence diet and/or weight and may include:
- What, when, how much eaten
- Activities during eating
- Emotions and cognitions related to meals/snacks
- Frequency, duration and intensity of exercise
- Target nutrient content of foods consumed (i.e., calories, fat, fiber)
- Event, thoughts about event, emotional response, behavioral response
- Negative self-talk, replacement thoughts
- Blood glucose, blood pressure

Self-monitoring is associated with improved treatment outcomes.

Implementation Tips
- Provide rationale and instructions for self-monitoring
- Review and identify patterns
- Assist with problem solving and goal setting
- Celebrate successes
- The amount of feedback required, typically diminishes as patient/client skill improves

STRATEGIES (C-2)

Problem solving
Techniques that are taught to assist clients in identifying barriers to achieving goals, identifying and implementing solutions and evaluating the effectiveness of the solutions.[2]

Implementation Tips
Work collaboratively with client to:
- Define the problem
- Brainstorm solutions
- Weigh pros/cons of potential solutions
- Select/implement strategy
- Evaluate outcomes
- Adjust strategy

Social support
Increased availability of social support for dietary behavior change. Social support may be generated among an individual's family, church, school, co-workers, health club or community.

Implementation Tips
A dietetics practitioner may assist a client by:
- Establishing a collaborative relationship
- Identifying family/community support
- Assisting clients in developing assertiveness skills.
- Utilize modeling, skill training, respondent and operant conditioning
- Conducting education in a group
- Encourage family involvement

Stress management
Reaction to stress can cause some clients to loss their appetite and others to overeat. Dietetics practitioners are particularly interested in management of stressful situations, which result in inappropriate eating behaviors.

Implementation Tips
Two approaches may be used to manage stress, one focuses on changing the environment, and the other focuses on modifying the client's response to stress.

Environmental-focused strategies may include:
- Guidance on planning ahead
- Use of time-management skills
- Developing a support system
- Building skills to prepare quick and healthful meals
- Guidance on eating on the run

Emotion-focused strategies may include:
- Use of positive self-talk
- Building assertiveness in expressing eating desires
- Setting realistic goals
- Learning to deal appropriately with emotion-driven eating cravings
- Relaxation exercises

COUNSELING

Edition: 2008

STRATEGIES (C-2)

Stimulus control

Identifying and modifying social or environmental cues or triggers to act, which encourage undesirable behaviors relevant to diet and exercise. In accordance with operant conditioning principles, attention is given to reinforcement and rewards.

Implementation Tips
- Review of self-monitoring records with clients may help to identify triggers for undesirable eating
- Assist client in identifying ways to modify the environment to eliminate triggers. This may include things such as:
  - Keeping food out of sight
  - Removing high sugar/high fat snacks from the house
  - Bringing lunch to work
  - Establishing a rule—no eating in the car
- Help client establish criteria for rewards for desirable behavior
- Ensure reward (reinforcement) received only if criteria met

Cognitive restructuring

Techniques used to increase client awareness of their perceptions of themselves and their beliefs related to diet, weight and weight loss expectations.

Implementation Tips
- Self-monitoring and techniques such as the ABC Technique of Irrational Beliefs may help clients to become more aware of thoughts that interfere in their ability to meet behavioral goals
- Help clients replace dysfunctional thoughts with more rationale ones
  - Challenge shoulds, oughts, musts
  - Decatastrophize expected outcomes
  - Confront faulty self-perceptions
  - Decenter by envisioning other perspectives
- Coach clients on replacing negative self-talk with more positive, empowering and affirming statements

Relapse prevention

Techniques used to help clients prepare to address high-risk situations for relapse with appropriate strategies and thinking. Incorporates both cognitive and behavioral strategies to enhance long-term behavior change outcomes.

Implementation Tips
Assist clients:
- Assess if external circumstances are contributing to lapse e.g., loss of job or support system
- Identify high-risk situations for slips
- Analyze reactions to slips
- Acquire knowledge and skills necessary to address high-risk situations
- Gain confidence in their ability to succeed in high-risk situations

COUNSELING

STRATEGIES (C-2)

Rewards/contingency management

A systematic process by which behaviors can be changed through the use of rewards for specific actions. Rewards may be derived from the client or the provider.

Implementation Tips

- Provide rewards for desired behaviors e.g., attendance, diet progress, consistent self-monitoring
- Rewards can be monetary, prizes, parking space, gift certificates
- Assist clients in determining rewards for achievement
- Ensure rewards are not received if progress is not made

COUNSELING

COORDINATION OF NUTRITION CARE DOMAIN

COORDINATION OF OTHER CARE DURING NUTRITION CARE (RC-1)

Definition

Facilitating services or interventions with other professionals, institutions, or agencies on behalf of the patient/client prior to discharge from nutrition care.

Details of Intervention

A typical intervention might be further described with the following details:

- Holding a team meeting to develop a comprehensive plan of care
- A formal referral for care by other dietetics practitioners who provide different expertise
- Collaboration with or referral to others such as the physician, dentist, physical therapist, social worker, occupational therapist, speech therapist, nurse, pharmacist, or other specialist dietitian
- Referral to an appropriate agency/program (e.g., home delivered meals, WIC, food pantry, soup kitchen, food stamps, housing assistance, shelters, rehabilitation, physical and mental disability programs, education training, and employment programs)

See reference manual for list of nutrition diagnoses, etiologies and signs and symptoms that often are associated with this intervention.

Other considerations (*e.g., patient/client negotiation, patient/client needs and desires, and readiness to change*)

- Availability of services related to patient/client need (specialty dietitians, clinical pharmacists, speech pathologists, nurse practitioners, etc.)
- Anticipated duration of health care encounter/hospital or long-term care discharge
- Resources available for care
- Medicare/Medicaid/insurance guidelines and restrictions
- Food assistance program (e.g., food stamp program) guidelines and regulations

COORDINATION

DISCHARGE AND TRANSFER OF NUTRITION CARE TO A NEW SETTING OR PROVIDER (RC-2)

Definition
Discharge planning and transfer of nutrition care from one level or location of care to another.

Details of Intervention
A typical intervention might be further described with the following details:
- Change in the nutrition prescription with consideration for changes in patient/client schedule, activity level, and food/nutrient availability in the new setting
- Collaboration with or referral to others such as the physician, dentist, physical therapist, social worker, occupational therapist, speech therapist, nurse, pharmacist, or other specialist dietitian
- Referral to an appropriate agency/program (e.g., home delivered meals, WIC, food pantry, soup kitchen, food stamps, housing assistance, shelters, rehabilitation, physical and mental disability programs, education, training and employment programs)

See reference manual for list of nutrition diagnoses, etiologies and signs and symptoms that often are associated with this intervention.

Other considerations (*e.g., patient/client negotiation, patient/client needs and desires, and readiness to change*)
- Availability of discharge planning services, options for care
- Preferences for the level and location of care
- Resources available for care
- Medicare/Medicaid/insurance guidelines and restrictions
- Health literacy
- Ability to implement treatment at home
- Food assistance program (e.g., food stamp program) guidelines and regulations

COORDINATION

Edition: 2008

SNAPshot
NCP Step 4. Nutrition Monitoring and Evaluation

What is the purpose of Nutrition Monitoring and Evaluation? The purpose is to determine the amount of progress made and if goals/expected outcomes are being met. Nutrition monitoring and evaluation identifies patient/client* outcomes relevant to the nutrition diagnosis and intervention plans and goals. Nutrition care outcomes—the desired results of nutrition care—are defined in this step. The change in specific nutrition care outcome indicators can be measured and compared to the patient/client's previous status, nutrition intervention goals, or reference standards. The aim is to promote more uniformity within the dietetics profession in assessing the effectiveness of nutrition intervention.

How does a dietetics practitioner determine what to measure for Nutrition Monitoring and Evaluation? Practitioners select nutrition care outcome indicators that will reflect a change as a result of nutrition care. In addition, dietetics practitioners will consider factors such as the nutrition diagnosis and its etiology and signs or symptoms, the nutrition intervention, medical diagnosis, health care outcome goals, quality management goals for nutrition, practice setting, patient/client population, and disease state and/or severity.

How are outcomes used in Nutrition Monitoring and Evaluation organized? In four categories.

Nutrition-Related Behavioral and Environmental Outcomes— *Nutrition-related knowledge, behavior, access, and ability that impact food and nutrient intake*

Food and Nutrient Intake Outcomes—*Food and/or nutrient intake from all sources*

Nutrition-Related Physical Sign and Symptom Outcomes— *Anthropometric, biochemical, and physical exam parameters*

Nutrition-Related Patient/Client-Centered Outcomes—*Perception of patient/client's nutrition intervention and its impact*

What does Nutrition Monitoring and Evaluation involve? Practitioners do three things as part of nutrition monitoring and evaluation—monitor, measure, and evaluate the changes in nutrition care indicators to determine patient/client progress. Practitioners *monitor* by providing evidence that the nutrition intervention is or is not changing the patient/client behavior or status. They *measure* outcomes by collecting data on the appropriate nutrition outcome indicator(s). Finally, dietetics practitioners compare the current findings with previous status, nutrition intervention goals, and/or reference standards (i.e., criteria) and *evaluate* the overall impact of the nutrition intervention on the patient's health outcomes. The use of standardized indicators and criteria increases the validity and reliability outcome data are collected. All these procedures facilitate electronic charting, coding, and outcomes measurement.

*Patient/client refers to individuals, groups, family members, and/or caregivers.

Are dietetics practitioners limited to the Nutrition Monitoring and Evaluation outcomes terms? A cascade of outcomes of nutrition care have been identified; each outcome has several possible indicators that can be measured depending on the patient/client population, practice setting, and disease state/severity. Dietetics practitioners can propose additions or revisions using the Procedure for Nutrition Controlled Vocabulary/Terminology Maintenance/Review available from ADA.

Detailed information about this step can be found in the International Dietetics and Nutrition Terminology (IDNT) Reference Manual: Standardized Language for the Nutrition Care Process, First Edition, American Dietetic Association.

Note: Clinical judgment must be used to select indicators and determine the appropriate measurement techniques and reference standards for a given patient population and setting. Once identified, these indicators, measurement techniques, and reference standards should be identified in policies and procedures or other documents for use in patient/client records, quality or performance improvement, or in formal research projects.

MONITOR & EVAL

BELIEFS AND ATTITUDES (BE-1.1)

Definition
Beliefs/attitudes about and/or readiness to change food, nutrition, or nutrition-related behaviors

Monitoring
Changes in these Potential Indicators:
- Readiness to change
- Perceived consequence of change
- Perceived costs versus benefits of change
- Perceived risk
- Outcome expectancy
- Conflict with personal/family value system
- Self-efficacy
  - o   Breastfeeding self-efficacy
  - o   Eating self-efficacy
  - o   Weight loss self-efficacy

Examples of the measurement methods or data sources for these outcome indicators
Patient/client self-report, client/patient assessment questionnaire or interview

Typically used to monitor and evaluate change in the following domains of nutrition interventions
Nutrition education, nutrition counseling

Typically used to monitor and evaluate change in the following nutrition diagnoses
Harmful beliefs/attitudes about food- or nutrition-related topics; not ready for diet/lifestyle change; inability to manage self-care; excess or inadequate oral food/beverage, energy, macronutrient, micronutrient or bioactive substance intake; imbalance of nutrients; inappropriate fat foods; inappropriate intake of amino acids; underweight; overweight/obesity; disordered eating pattern; physical inactivity; excess exercise.

BEHAVIORAL

BELIEFS AND ATTITUDES (BE-1.1)

Evaluation

Criteria for evaluation
Comparison to Goal or Reference Standard:
1. Goal (tailored to individual's needs)
OR
2. Reference standard

Patient/Client Example(s)
Example(s) of one or two of the Nutrition Care Indicators for this outcome (*includes sample initial and re-assessment documentation for one of the indicators*)

Indicator(s) selected
Readiness to change

Criteria for evaluation
Comparison to Goal or Reference Standard:
1. Goal: Patient/client is currently in the precontemplation stage of change. Intervention goal is to move patient to the contemplation stage of change (recognition of the need to change) within 3 months.
OR
2. Reference standard: No validated standard exists.

Sample monitoring and evaluation documentation

Initial encounter with patient/ client	Assessment results indicate patient/client is currently in the precontemplation stage of change related to need for DASH diet adherence. Will reassess in eight weeks.
Re-assessment after nutrition intervention	Reassessment indicates that patient/client has moved from the precontemplation stage to the contemplation stage related to need for DASH diet adherence. Will reassess in eight weeks.

Suggested references for indicators, measurement techniques, and reference standards are available in the International Dietetics and Nutrition Terminology (IDNT) Reference Manual.

BEHAVIORAL

Edition: 2008

FOOD AND NUTRITION KNOWLEDGE (BE-1.2)

Definition
Level of knowledge about food, nutrition and health, or nutrition-related information and guidelines relevant to patient/client needs

Monitoring
Changes in these Potential Indicators:
- Level of knowledge (e.g., none, limited, minimal, substantial, and extensive)
- Areas of knowledge
    - o Food/nutrient requirements
    - o Physiological functions
    - o Disease/condition
    - o Nutrition recommendations
    - o Food products
    - o Consequences of food behavior
    - o Food label understanding/knowledge
    - o Self-management parameters

NOTE: There are two dimensions of knowledge: level and area.

Examples of the measurement methods or data sources for this outcome
Pre- and/or post-tests administered orally, on paper or by computer, scenario discussions, patient/client restate key information, review of food records, practical demonstration/test

Typically used to monitor and evaluate change in the following domains of nutrition interventions
Nutrition education, nutrition counseling

Typically used to monitor and evaluate change in the following nutrition diagnoses
Food- and nutrition-related knowledge deficit, limited adherence to nutrition-related recommendations, intake domain

BEHAVIORAL

FOOD AND NUTRITION KNOWLEDGE (BE-1.2)

Evaluation

Criteria for evaluation
Comparison to Goal or Reference Standard:
1. Goal (tailored to individual's needs)
   OR
2. Reference standard

Patient/Client Example(s)

Example(s) of one or two of the Nutrition Care Indicators for this outcome (*includes sample initial and re-assessment documentation for one of the indicators*)

Indicator(s) selected
Area of knowledge (carbohydrate counting)

Criteria for evaluation
Comparison to Goal or Reference Standard:
1. Goal: Patient/client will be able to accurately read a food label and identify the total number of grams of carbohydrate per serving.
   OR
2. Reference standard: No validated standard exists.

Sample monitoring and evaluation documentation

Initial encounter with patient/ client	Patient/client with newly diagnosed diabetes with limited knowledge regarding carbohydrate counting.
Re-assessment after nutrition intervention	Patient/client with moderate knowledge regarding carbohydrate counting. Able to apply knowledge to common scenarios, but not consistently able to apply knowledge to solve problems. Will continue to monitor at next encounter in one week.

Suggested references for indicators, measurement techniques, and reference standards are available in the International Dietetics and Nutrition Terminology (IDNT) Reference Manual.

BEHAVIORAL

Edition: 2008

ABILITY TO PLAN MEALS/SNACKS (BE-2.1)

Definition
Patient/client ability level related to planning healthy meals and snacks, which are compatible with dietary goals

Monitoring
Change in this Potential Indicator:
- Meal/snack planning ability (e.g., may include ability to use planning tools, plan a menu, create/tailor a meal plan, create/use a shopping list)

Examples of the measurement methods or data sources for these outcome indicators
Food intake records, self-report or caregiver report, 24-hour recall, menu review, targeted questionnaire

Typically used to measure the outcomes for the following domains of nutrition interventions
Nutrition education, nutrition counseling

Typically used to monitor and evaluate change in the following nutrition diagnosis
Excessive or inadequate oral food/beverage intake, underweight, overweight/obesity, limited adherence to nutrition related recommendations, inability or lack of desire to manage self-care

Evaluation

Criteria for evaluation
Comparison to Goal or Reference Standard:
1. Goal (tailored to individual's needs)
OR
2. Reference standard

BEHAVIORAL

ABILITY TO PLAN MEALS/SNACKS (BE-2.1)

Patient/Client Example(s)

Example(s) of one or two of the Nutrition Care Indicators for this outcome (*includes sample initial and re-assessment documentation for one of the indicators*)

Indicator(s) selected

Meal/snack planning ability (e.g., may include ability to use planning tools, plan a menu, create/tailor a meal plan, create/use a shopping list)

Criteria for evaluation

Comparison to Goal or Reference Standard:
1. Goal: Patient/client states that lack of planning impedes her progress. Patient/client currently never preplans meals/snacks and set a goal to develop or tailor a meal plan and follow it 6 days per week.

OR

2. Reference standard: No validated standard exists.

Sample monitoring and evaluation documentation

Initial encounter with patient/ client	Patient/client states that lack of planning is a barrier to success. She rated herself a 2 on a scale of 1-10 on her ability to plan meals/snacks. Patient/client set goal to develop a meal plan prior to the beginning of each week. Will assess meal-planning skill at next encounter in two weeks.
Re-assessment after nutrition intervention	Significant progress made toward goal. Patient/client rated herself an 8 on a scale of 1-10 on her ability to plan meals at the beginning of each week. She tailored a meal plan she found in a magazine to her family's lifestyle. Patient/client would like to add more variety at the dinner meal. Will continue to monitor patient/client goal to preplan meals at next encounter in two weeks.

Suggested references for indicators, measurement techniques, and reference standards are available in the International Dietetics and Nutrition Terminology (IDNT) Reference Manual.

BEHAVIORAL

Edition: 2008

ABILITY TO SELECT HEALTHFUL FOOD/MEALS (BE-2.2)

Definition
Patient/client ability level related to making selections at food stores and/or restaurants that are compatible with dietary goals

Monitoring
Change in this Potential Indicator:
- Food/meal selection (e.g., may include ability to do the following: Interpret food labels, select healthful menu items, select healthful versions of food items, tailor/modify portion sizes)

Examples of the measurement methods or data sources for these outcome indicators
Food intake records, self-report or caregiver report, 24-hour recall, food frequency questionnaire, menu analysis, targeted questionnaires and monitoring devices

Typically used to measure the outcomes for the following domains of nutrition interventions
Nutrition education, nutrition counseling

Typically used to monitor and evaluate change in the following nutrition diagnosis
Excessive or inadequate oral food/beverage intake, overweight/obesity, disordered eating pattern, undesirable food choices, limited adherence to nutrition related recommendations, inability or lack of desire to manage self-care

Evaluation

Criteria for evaluation:
Comparison to Goal or Reference Standard:
1. Goal (tailored to individual's needs)
   OR
2. Reference standard

BEHAVIORAL

ABILITY TO SELECT HEALTHFUL FOOD/MEALS (BE-2.2)

Patient/Client Example(s)

Example(s) of one or two of the Nutrition Care Indicators for this outcome (*includes sample initial and re-assessment documentation for one of the indicators*)

Indicator(s) selected

Food/meal selection (e.g., may include ability to do the following: Interpret food labels, select healthful menu items, select healthful versions of food items, tailor/ modify portion sizes)

Criteria for evaluation:

Comparison to Goal or Reference Standard:

1. Goal: Patient/client currently selects high-fat entrees at lunch 5 days per week and has a goal of selecting low-fat entrees at lunch 5 day per week.

OR

2. Reference standard: No validated standard exists.

Sample monitoring and evaluation documentation

Initial encounter with patient/ client	Based on patient/client food diary, patient/client consuming high-fat entrees at lunch 5 days/week. Will monitor quality of food selections at lunch at next encounter in one week.
Re-assessment at a later date	Some progress toward goal. Based upon lunch diary, patient/ client selected low-fat entrees 3 of 5 days. Will continue to monitor quality of lunch menu selections.

Suggested references for indicators, measurement techniques, and reference standards are available in the International Dietetics and Nutrition Terminology (IDNT) Reference Manual.

BEHAVIORAL

Edition: 2008

ABILITY TO PREPARE HEALTHFUL FOOD/MEALS (BE-2.3)

Definition

Patient/client ability level related to preparing food and meals that are compatible with dietary goals

Monitoring

Change in this Potential Indicator:

- Food/meal preparation ability (e.g., may include meat, grain/starch, vegetable preparation, dinner preparation, recipe modification, recipe implementation)

Examples of the measurement methods or data sources for these outcome indicators
Food intake records, self-report or caregiver report, 24-hour recall, menu review, targeted questionnaire

Typically used to measure the outcomes for the following domains of nutrition interventions
Nutrition education, nutrition counseling

Typically used to monitor and evaluate change in the following nutrition diagnosis
Impaired ability to prepare foods/meals, excessive or inadequate oral food/beverage intake, underweight, overweight/obesity, limited adherence to nutrition related recommendations, inability or lack of desire to manage self-care

Evaluation

Criteria for evaluation:
Comparison to Goal or Reference Standard:
1. Goal (tailored to individual's needs)
OR
2. Reference standard

BEHAVIORAL

ABILITY TO PREPARE HEALTHFUL FOOD/MEALS (BE-2.3)

Patient/Client Example(s)

Example(s) of one or two of the Nutrition Care Indicators for this outcome (*includes sample initial and re-assessment documentation for one of the indicators*)

Indicator(s) selected

Food/meal preparation ability (e.g., may include meat, grain/starch, vegetable preparation; dinner preparation; recipe modification; recipe implementation)

Comparison to Goal or Reference Standard

1. Goal: Patient/client states that she does not know how to prepare vegetables so her family will eat them. Set goal to try three new ways to prepare vegetables, which may be acceptable to her family.

   OR

2. Reference standard: No validated standard exists.

Sample monitoring and evaluation documentation

Initial encounter with patient/ client	Patient/client states that she is unable prepare vegetables in a healthy way (not fried) acceptable to herself and her family. She set goal to try three new techniques or recipes for vegetable preparation this week. Will monitor vegetable preparation skill at next encounter in two weeks.
Re-assessment after nutrition intervention	Some progress made. Patient/client tried one new recipe for preparing vegetables and it was highly acceptable to family. Will continue to monitor patient/client's goal to try new vegetable preparation techniques at next encounter in two weeks.

Suggested references for indicators, measurement techniques, and reference standards are available in the International Dietetics and Nutrition Terminology (IDNT) Reference Manual.

BEHAVIORAL

Edition: 2008

ADHERENCE (BE-2.4)

Definition

Level of compliance with nutrition-related recommendations or behavioral changes agreed upon by patient/client to achieve nutrition-related goals

Monitoring

Changes in these Potential Indicators:
- Self-reported adherence score
- Biochemical marker for adherence

NOTE: Use in conjunction with appropriate outcomes from Food and Nutrition Intake and Nutrition-Related Sign/Symptom outcome domains. May be useful in relapse prevention treatment (analyze and control factors that caused the lapse).

Examples of the measurement methods or data sources for these outcome indicators

Attendance, self-monitoring records, patient/client self-report, adherence tools or questionnaires, provider assessment

Typically used to measure the outcomes for the following domains of nutrition interventions

Food and/or nutrient delivery, nutrition education, nutrition counseling

Typically used to monitor and evaluate change in the following nutrition diagnosis

Limited adherence to nutrition-related recommendations

Evaluation

Criteria for evaluation

Comparison to Goal or Reference Standard:
1. Goal (tailored to individual's needs)
OR
2. Reference standard

BEHAVIORAL

ADHERENCE (BE-2.4)

Patient/Client Example(s)

Example(s) of one or two of the Nutrition Care Indicators for this outcome (*includes sample initial and re-assessment documentation for one of the indicators*)

Indicator(s) selected
Self-reported adherence score

Criteria for evaluation
Comparison to Goal or Reference Standard:

1. Goal: Patient/client rates herself a 4 on a scale of 1 to 10 (1 meaning never and 10 meaning always) on her level of compliance with nutrition-related goals. Patient/client desires to get self to a rating of 8.

    OR

2. Reference standard: No validated standard exists.

Sample monitoring and evaluation documentation

Initial encounter with patient/ client	Patient/client rates herself a 1 on a scale of 1-10 on her ability to adhere to her meal plan. Patient/client set a goal to adhere to her meal plan 5 days per week. Will evaluate adherence at the next encounter.
Re-assessment after nutrition intervention	Some progress toward goal. Patient/client rated herself a 6 on a scale of 1-10 on her ability to meet her adherence goal of following her meal plan 5 days per week. Is doing well on weekdays, but states she must improve on weekends. Will monitor at next encounter in two weeks.

Suggested references for indicators, measurement techniques, and reference standards are available in the International Dietetics and Nutrition Terminology (IDNT) Reference Manual.

BEHAVIORAL

Edition: 2008

GOAL SETTING (BE-2.5)

Definition

Patient/client ability level related to setting specific, realistic (in light of current skill level and beliefs), positive goals pertinent to food- and nutrition-related behaviors

Monitoring

Changes in these Potential Indicators:

- Goal setting ability (e.g., may include the ability to set specific, measurable, attainable, realistic, time-sensitive goals)

Examples of the measurement methods or data sources for these outcome indicators
Self-monitoring records, client/patient self-report, goal tracking tools

Typically used to monitor and evaluate change in the following domains of nutrition interventions
Nutrition education, nutrition counseling

Typically used to monitor and evaluate change in the following nutrition diagnosis
Excess oral food/beverage intake, excess or inadequate energy, macronutrient, micronutrient or bioactive substance intake, overweight/obesity, disordered eating pattern, inability or lack of desire to manage self-care, limited adherence to nutrition-related recommendations

Evaluation

Criteria for evaluation
Comparison to Goal or Reference Standard:
1. Goal (tailored to individual's needs)
OR
2. Reference standard

BEHAVIORAL

GOAL SETTING (BE-2.5)

Patient/Client Example(s)

Example(s) of one or two of the Nutrition Care Indicators for this outcome (*includes sample initial and re-assessment documentation for one of the indicators*)

Indicator(s) selected

Goal setting ability (e.g., may include the ability to set specific, measurable, attainable, realistic, time-sensitive goals)

Criteria for evaluation

Comparison to Goal or Reference Standard:

1. Goal: Patient/Client's current goal is to loss 30 pounds in 8 weeks. Following counseling, patient/client will be able to define a realistic weight loss goal and behavioral steps to achieve that long-term goal.

   OR

2. Reference standard: No validated standard exists.

Sample monitoring and evaluation documentation

Initial encounter with patient/ client	Patient/client frequently sets unrealistic goals and verbalizes frustration. Current goal is to loss 30 pounds in 8 weeks with no clear strategy.
Re-assessment after nutrition intervention	Some progress toward goal. Patient/client set goal to limit sweets to 1 serving/day and lose two pounds per week. Will continue to assess goal-setting skill at next encounter in two weeks.

Suggested references for indicators, measurement techniques, and reference standards are available in the International Dietetics and Nutrition Terminology (IDNT) Reference Manual.

BEHAVIORAL

Edition: 2008

PORTION CONTROL (BE-2.6)

Definition
Patient/client ability level related to selecting and eating appropriate quantities of food (portion sizes) for a meal or snack, compatible with dietary goals

Monitoring
Changes in these Potential Indicators:
- Portion size eaten

Examples of the measurement methods or data sources for these outcome indicators
Food intake records, 24 hour recall, observation, response to questionnaire or interview questions

Typically used to monitor and evaluate change in the following domains of nutrition interventions
Food and/or nutrient delivery, nutrition education, nutrition counseling

Typically used to monitor and evaluate change in the following nutrition diagnoses
Excess or inadequate oral food/beverage intake, excess or inadequate energy, macronutrient, micronutrient or bioactive substance intake, imbalance of nutrients, inappropriate intake of types of carbohydrate, inconsistent carbohydrate intake, inappropriate fat foods, inappropriate intake of amino acids, underweight, overweight/obesity, disordered eating pattern, inability or lack of desire to manage self-care

Evaluation

Criteria for evaluation
Comparison to Goal or Reference Standard:
1. Goal (tailored to individual's needs): Compare progress to patient's baseline.
OR
2. Reference standard

PORTION CONTROL (BE-2.6)

Patient/Client Example(s)

Example(s) of one or two of the Nutrition Care Indicators for this outcome (*includes sample initial and re-assessment documentation for one of the indicators*)

Indicator(s) selected
Portion size eaten

Criteria for evaluation
Comparison to Goal or Reference Standard:
1. Nutrition prescription or goal: Patient/client eats out for lunch 5 days per week and consumes all food served. Patient/client goal is to ask restaurant server to serve a half portion of the entrée and wrap the remainder to take home.

OR

2. Reference standard: No validated standard exists.

Sample monitoring and evaluation documentation

Initial encounter with patient/ client	Patient/client identified portion control as a significant diet problem. Discussed portion control strategies and will monitor patient/client's success in implementing these at the next encounter.
Re-assessment after nutrition intervention	Significant progress toward goal. Patient/client rated herself a 6 on a scale of 1-10 on her ability to control portions. Is doing well at home, but states she must do better at restaurants. Discussed strategies that may be helpful at restaurants. Will monitor at next encounter in two weeks.

Suggested references for indicators, measurement techniques, and reference standards are available in the International Dietetics and Nutrition Terminology (IDNT) Reference Manual.

BEHAVIORAL

Edition: 2008

SELF-CARE MANAGEMENT (BE-2.7)

Definition
Alteration in ability to make judgments and implement action on a day-to-day basis to control a nutrition-related condition.

Monitoring
Changes in these Potential Indicators:
- Self-care management ability (e.g., may include interpreting results, problem solving, initiating appropriate action,symptom management and emergency prevention)

NOTE: Self-monitoring ability is covered on Self-Monitoring Reference Sheet.

Examples of the measurement methods or data sources for these outcome indicators
Client/patient self-report, caregiver report, self-care management tools, lab values, weight, ability to demonstrate using a scenario

Typically used to measure the outcomes for the following domains of nutrition interventions
Nutrition education, nutrition counseling

Typically used to monitor and evaluate change in the following nutrition diagnosis
Inability or lack of desire to manage self-care, excessive oral food/beverage intake, excess energy intake, excess macronutrient and micronutrient intake, involuntary weight loss, poor nutrition quality of life, self-feeding difficulty

Evaluation

Criteria for evaluation
Comparison to Goal or Reference Standard:
1. Goal (tailored to individual's needs)
OR
2. Reference standard

SELF-CARE MANAGEMENT (BE-2.7)

Patient/Client Example(s)

Example(s) of one or two of the Nutrition Care Indicators for this outcome (*includes sample initial and re-assessment documentation for one of the indicators*)

Indicator(s) selected

Self-care management ability (e.g., may include interpreting results, problem solving, initiating appropriate action, symptom management and emergency prevention)

Criteria for evaluation

Comparison to Goal or Reference Standard:

1. Goal: Patient/Client with diabetes reaching stage to accept greater responsibility in self-management of type 1 diabetes. Patient to monitor blood glucose and adjust carbohydrate intake at lunch and meals away from home.
OR
2. Reference standard: No validated standard exists.

Sample monitoring and evaluation documentation

Initial encounter with patient/ client	Patient/client states that he has not participated in diabetes self-care management in the past and rates himself a 1 on a scale of 1-10 on his ability to do self-care management. Patient/client set goal to monitoring blood glucose and adjust carbohydrate intake in the afternoons, 5 days per week. Will evaluate self-care management skill at the next encounter.
Re-assessment after nutrition intervention	Some progress toward goal. Patient/client rated himself a 5, on a scale of 1-10, on his ability to meet his self-care management goal of monitoring blood glucose and adjusting carbohydrate intake in the afternoon, 5 days per week. Is doing well on weekdays, but states he must do better on weekends. Will monitor at next encounter in two weeks.

Suggested references for indicators, measurement techniques, and reference standards are available in the International Dietetics and Nutrition Terminology (IDNT) Reference Manual.

BEHAVIORAL

Edition: 2008

SELF-MONITORING (BE-2.8)

Definition
Ability level related to using techniques to observe and document feelings, behaviors, weight or blood/urine values to achieve a goal

Monitoring
Changes in these Potential Indicators:
- Self-monitoring ability (e.g., may include completeness of monitoring and frequency of monitoring)

NOTE: Application of self-monitoring information is covered on Self-Care Management Reference Sheet.

Examples of the measurement methods or data sources for these outcome indicators
Food diaries/records, weight records, blood glucose monitoring, physical activity record, behavior checklists

Typically used to measure the outcomes for the following domains of nutrition interventions
Nutrition education, nutrition counseling

Typically used to monitor and evaluate change in the following nutrition diagnoses
Underweight, overweight/obesity, disordered eating pattern, undesirable food choices, physical inactivity, inability or lack of desire to manage self-care, self-monitoring deficit, not ready for lifestyle change, limited adherence, excessive exercise

Evaluation

Criteria for evaluation
Comparison to Goal or Reference Standard:
1. Goal (tailored to individual's needs)
OR
2. Reference standard

BEHAVIORAL

SELF-MONITORING (BE-2.8)

Patient/Client Example(s)

Example(s) of one or two of the Nutrition Care Indicators for this outcome (*includes sample initial and re-assessment documentation for one of the indicators*)

Indicator(s) selected

Self-monitoring ability (e.g., may include completeness of monitoring and frequency of monitoring)

Criteria for evaluation

Comparison to Goal or Reference Standard:

1. Goal: Patient/client enrolled in lifestyle change program and has never kept a food diary. Patient/client goal is to maintain a food intake record 5 days per week recording time, food, portion size, calorie and fat content.

OR

2. Reference standard: No validated standard exists.

Sample monitoring and evaluation documentation

Initial encounter with patient/ client	Based upon patient/client records, patient/client monitoring blood glucose 1 day/wk and is not monitoring carbohydrate intake. Will evaluate blood glucose and carbohydrate counting records at the next encounter.
Re-assessment after nutrition intervention	Some progress toward self-monitoring goal. Patient/client recording blood glucose levels 2 day/wk and carbohydrate intake 2 times/week. Will continue to monitor self-monitoring at next encounter in 2 weeks.

Suggested references for indicators, measurement techniques, and reference standards are available in the International Dietetics and Nutrition Terminology (IDNT) Reference Manual.

Edition: 2008

BEHAVIORAL

SOCIAL SUPPORT (BE-2.9)

Definition
Ability level related to building and utilizing a network of family, friends, colleagues, health professionals, and community resources for encouragement, emotional support and enhancing environment to support behavior change

Monitoring
Changes in these Potential Indicators:
- Ability to build and utilize social support (e.g., may include perceived social support, social integration, and assertiveness)

Examples of the measurement methods or data sources for these outcome indicators
Self-monitoring records, client/patient self-report, goal tracking tools

Typically used to monitor and evaluate change in the following domains of nutrition interventions Nutrition counseling

Typically used to monitor and evaluate change in the following nutrition diagnosis
Intake domain, underweight, overweight/obesity, disordered eating pattern, undesirable food choices, inability or lack of desire to manage self-care, breastfeeding difficulty, not ready for diet/lifestyle change, limited adherence to nutrition-related recommendations

Evaluation

Criteria for evaluation
Comparison to Goal or Reference Standard:
1. Goal (tailored to individual's needs)
OR
2. Reference standard

SOCIAL SUPPORT (BE-2.9)

Patient/Client Example(s)

Example(s) of one or two of the Nutrition Care Indicators for this outcome (*includes sample initial and re-assessment documentation for one of the indicators*)

Indicator(s) selected

Ability to build and utilize social support (e.g., may include perceived social support, social integration, and assertiveness)

Criteria for evaluation

Comparison to Goal or Reference Standard:
1. Goal: Overweight patient/client's wife adds fat to all foods prepared at home. Goal is reduce the amount of fat in meals prepared at home by asking wife to not dress the salad or add fat seasoning to vegetables before serving.
   OR
2. Reference standard: No validated standard exists.

Sample monitoring and evaluation documentation

Initial encounter with patient/client	Patient/client states that he rarely verbalizes his nutrition-related desires/needs in family or social situations and rates his ability to elicit social support a 3 on a scale of 1 to 10. Will evaluate at the next encounter.
Re-assessment at a later date	Some progress toward goal. Patient/client rated himself a 5, on a scale of 1-10, on his ability to elicit social support. Has begun to verbalize his needs and plans to research restaurants that meet his needs that others will enjoy. Will monitor at next encounter in two weeks.

Suggested references for indicators, measurement techniques, and reference standards are available in the International Dietetics and Nutrition Terminology (IDNT) Reference Manual.

BEHAVIORAL

Edition: 2008

STIMULUS CONTROL (BE-2.10)

Definition
Ability level related to developing/implementing strategies to manage eating behavior and physical activity in response to stimuli

Monitoring
Changes in these Potential Indicators:
- Ability to manage behavior in response to stimuli (e.g., may include ability to identify triggers/cues, develop a plan, modify environment or behavior)

Examples of the measurement methods or data sources for these outcome indicators
Self-monitoring records, client/patient self-report

Typically used to monitor and evaluate change in the following domains of nutrition interventions
Nutrition education, nutrition counseling

Typically used to monitor and evaluate change in the following nutrition diagnosis
Excess oral food/beverage, energy, macronutrient or bioactive substance intake; imbalance of nutrients; inappropriate intake of types of carbohydrate; inconsistent carbohydrate intake; inappropriate fat foods; underweight; overweight/obesity; disordered eating pattern; undesirable food choices; inability or lack of desire to manage self-care; physical inactivity; excess exercise

Evaluation

Criteria for evaluation
Comparison to Goal or Reference Standard:
1. Goal (tailored to individual's needs)
OR
2. Reference standard

BEHAVIORAL

STIMULUS CONTROL (BE-2.10)

Patient/Client Example(s)

Example(s) of one or two of the Nutrition Care Indicators for this outcome (*includes sample initial and re-assessment documentation for one of the indicators*)

Indicator(s) selected

Ability to build and utilize social support (e.g., may include perceived social support, social integration, and assertiveness)

Criteria for evaluation

Comparison to Goal or Reference Standard:

1. Goal: After monitoring behavior using a self-monitoring record, patient becomes aware that she is over eating while watching the 10 PM news and realizes every time the TV is on she feels hungry. She sets a goal to no longer eat while watching TV.

OR

2. Reference standard: No validated standard exists.

Sample monitoring and evaluation documentation

Initial encounter with patient/ client	Based upon self-monitoring, patient/client identified that she eats while watching TV, 7 days per week and desires to eliminate the TV as a trigger for inappropriate eating. Patient/ client currently rates herself a 2, on a scale of 1–10 on ability to manage eating while watching TV (trigger). Will monitor patient/client's achievement of goal at next encounter in one week.
Re-assessment after nutrition intervention	Met stimulus control goal. Patient/client rated herself a 9 on a scale of 1-10 on ability to eat appropriately while watching TV. She has started using the treadmill and knitting in front of the TV rather than eating. Will continue to monitor progress over the next few weeks to ensure sustainment of behavior change.

Suggested references for indicators, measurement techniques, and reference standards are available in the International Dietetics and Nutrition Terminology (IDNT) Reference Manual.

BEHAVIORAL

Edition: 2008

ACCESS TO A SUFFICIENT, RELIABLE SUPPLY OF SAFE, HEALTHFUL FOOD (BE-3.1.1)

Definition

Degree to which enough healthful, safe food is available

Monitoring

Changes in these Potential Indicators:

- Access to a sufficient supply of healthful food
  (e.g., access to federal programs, such as, WIC and the Food Stamp Program and/or community programs, such as food pantries and meal sites; access to financial resources, school/community food programs with healthful food choices, and/or to transportation; assistance in securing food; caregiver support and access to food; participation in federal and/or community food programs)
- Access to safe food
  (e.g., procurement, identification of safe food, preparation and/or storage techniques)

Examples of the measurement methods or data sources for these outcome indicators
Patient/client report overall food availability/food consumed during the week, referral information, home evaluation

Typically used to measure the outcomes for the following domains of nutrition interventions
Nutrition education, nutrition counseling, coordination of nutrition care

Typically used to monitor and evaluate change in the following nutrition diagnoses
Access to food, access to safe food, inadequate or excessive energy intake

Evaluation

Criteria for evaluation
Comparison to Goal or Reference Standard:
1. Goal (tailored to patient/client needs)
OR
2. Reference standard

ACCESS TO A SUFFICIENT, RELIABLE SUPPLY OF SAFE, HEALTHFUL FOOD (BE-3.1.1)

Patient/Client Example(s)

Example(s) of one or two of the Nutrition Care Indicators for this outcome (*includes sample initial and re-assessment documentation for one of the indicators*)

Indicator(s) selected

Access to a sufficient supply of healthful food

Criteria for evaluation

Comparison to Goal or Reference Standard:

1. Goal: Patient/client has limited access to a sufficient quantity of food when substantial or extensive access to a sufficient, reliable supply of food is the goal.

   OR

2. Reference standard: No validated standard exists.

Sample monitoring and evaluation documentation

Initial encounter with patient/ client	The patient/client has limited access to a sufficient, reliable supply of food. Will monitor change in access to food at next appointment.
Re-assessment after nutrition intervention	Some progress toward goal as patient/client has moderate access to a sufficient, reliable supply of food.

Suggested references for indicators, measurement techniques, and reference standards are available in the International Dietetics and Nutrition Terminology (IDNT) Reference Manual.

BEHAVIORAL

Edition: 2008

BREASTFEEDING SUCCESS (BE-4.1)

Definition

Degree to which breastfeeding plans and experience meet nutritional and other needs of the infant and mother

Monitoring

Changes in these Potential Indicators:

- Initiation of breastfeeding
- Duration of breastfeeding
- Exclusive breastfeeding
- Breastfeeding problems

NOTE: Infant/child growth can be found on the Body Composition/Growth Reference Sheet. Breastfeeding self-efficacy and intention to breastfeed can be found on the Beliefs and Attitudes Reference Sheet.

Examples of the measurement methods or data sources for these outcome indicators
Patient/client report, practitioner observation of breastfeeding dyad, self-monitoring records, infant weight trends

Typically used to measure the outcomes for the following domains of nutrition interventions
Nutrition education, nutrition counseling, coordination of nutrition care

Typically used to monitor and evaluate change in the following nutrition diagnoses
Maternal breastfeeding difficulty, food- and nutrition-related knowledge deficit, harmful beliefs/attitudes about food- or nutrition-related topics; and infant underweight, involuntary weight loss, inadequate fluid intake

BEHAVIORAL

BREASTFEEDING SUCCESS (BE-4.1)

Evaluation

Criteria for evaluation
Comparison to Goal or Reference Standard:
1. Goal (tailored to patient/client's needs)
OR
2. Reference standard

Patient/Client Example(s)
Example(s) of one or two of the Nutrition Care Indicators for this outcome (*includes sample initial and re-assessment documentation for one of the indicators*)

Indicator(s) selected
Initiation of breastfeeding

Criteria for evaluation
Comparison to Goal or Reference Standard:
1. Goal: Patient/client currently fears her breast milk supply is not adequate and worries about how she will manage when she returns to work in four weeks. Goal is for mother to breastfeed for six months.
OR
2. Reference standard: No validated standard exists.

Sample monitoring and evaluation documentation

Initial encounter with patient/ client	Postpartum patient/client states she is planning to use a combination of formula and breastfeed and start solids at 3 months. Will educate and refer to lactation support group.
Re-assessment after nutrition intervention	Patient/client reports she has exclusively breast fed for three months and plans to delay introduction of solids. Will reinforce and educate. Continue to monitor.

Suggested references for indicators, measurement techniques, and reference standards are available in the International Dietetics and Nutrition Terminology (IDNT) Reference Manual.

BEHAVIORAL

Edition: 2008

NUTRITION-RELATED ACTIVITIES OF DAILY LIVING AND INSTRUMENTAL ACTIVITIES OF DAILY LIVING (BE-4.2)

Definition
Level of cognitive and physical ability to perform nutrition-related activities of daily living and instrumental activities of daily living by older and/or disabled persons

Monitoring
Changes in these Potential Indicators:
- Acceptance of assistance with eating
- Ability to use adaptive eating devices
- Time taken to eat and consume meals
- Ability to shop for food
- Nutrition-related activities of daily living (ADL) score
- Nutrition-related instrumental activities of daily living (IADL) score

NOTE: Sufficient intake of food can be found on the Food Intake Reference Sheet. Sufficient intake of fluid can be found on the Fluid/Beverage Intake Reference Sheet. Food security and ability to maintain sanitation can be found on the Access to Food Reference Sheet. Ability to prepare/cook food can be found on the Ability to Prepare Healthy Food/Meals Reference Sheet.

Examples of the measurement methods or data sources for these outcome indicators
Self-report, caregiver report, home visit, targeted questionnaires and monitoring devices, ADL and/or IADL measurement tool, congregate meal site attendance records

Typically used to monitor and evaluate change in the following domains of nutrition interventions Coordination of nutrition care

Typically used to monitor and evaluate change in the following nutrition diagnoses
Inability to manage self-care, impaired ability to prepare foods/meals

NUTRITION-RELATED ACTIVITIES OF DAILY LIVING AND INSTRUMENTAL ACTIVITIES OF DAILY LIVING (BE-4.2)

Evaluation

Criteria for evaluation

Comparison to Goal or Reference Standard:
1. Goal (tailored to patient/client's needs)
OR
2. Reference standard

Patient/Client Example(s)

Example(s) of one or two of the Nutrition Care Indicators for this outcome (*includes sample initial and re-assessment documentation for one of the indicators*)

Indicator(s) selected

Nutrition-related instrumental activities of daily living (IADL) score

Criteria for evaluation

Comparison to Goal or Reference Standard:
1. Goal: Patient/client with decreased food intake because of impaired ability to use eating utensils sets goal to utilize adaptive eating devices at meals to decrease eating difficulty.
OR
2. Reference standard: No validated standard exists.

Sample monitoring and evaluation documentation

Initial encounter with patient/ client	Patient/client with inadequate food intake due to inability to drive, no close relative living in vicinity, subsequent weight loss and difficulties in performing ADLs and IADLs due to weakness. Client is to use new strategies and community resources to facilitate attendance at senior center congregate meals 5 times per week, use of community provided transportation offered to grocery store 1 x per week and attendance in strength training at senior center.
Re-assessment after nutrition intervention	Significant progress in nutrition-related activities of daily living. Patient/client able to attend senior center for meals and strength training 3 times this week. Goal is 5 times. Will continue to assess at next encounter. Client going to grocery store 1 x per week.

Suggested references for indicators, measurement techniques, and reference standards are available in the International Dietetics and Nutrition Terminology (IDNT) Reference Manual.

BEHAVIORAL

Edition: 2008

PHYSICAL ACTIVITY (BE-4.3)

Definition
Level of physical activity and/or amount of exercise performed

Monitoring
Changes in these Potential Indicators:
- Consistency/frequency
- Duration
- Intensity
- Strength

Examples of the measurement methods or data sources for these outcome indicators
Exercise log, watch, pedometer with a time function, and other electronic monitoring devices that detect time and intensity; attendance at strength training, balance training (for older adults), and/or aerobic classes

Typically used to measure the outcomes for the following domains of nutrition interventions
Nutrition education, nutrition counseling

Typically used to monitor and evaluate change in the following nutrition diagnoses
Physical inactivity, excessive exercise, underweight, overweight/obesity, involuntary weight loss or weight gain

Evaluation

Criteria for evaluation
Comparison to Goal or Reference Standard:
1. Goal (tailored to patient/client's needs)
OR
2. Reference standard

BEHAVIORAL

PHYSICAL ACTIVITY (BE-4.3)

Patient/Client Example(s)

Example(s) of one or two of the Nutrition Care Indicators for this outcome (*includes sample initial and re-assessment documentation for one of the indicators*)

Indicator(s) selected
Consistency and duration

Criteria for evaluation
Comparison to Goal or Reference Standard:
1. Goal: Patient/client is currently completely sedentary, but established a goal to walk 10 minutes per day, 6 days per week.
   OR
2. Reference standard: Patient/client's typical 10-minute walk, twice a week is well below the recommended 30 minutes of moderate-intensity physical activity, but above usual activity, at work or home most days/wk (Dietary Guidelines for Americans 2005).

Sample monitoring and evaluation documentation

Initial encounter with patient/ client	Based upon exercise log, patient/client doing moderate-intensity physical activities 30 minutes/day, 2 days/week. Goal is to exercise 30 minutes/day, moderate-intensity activities, 5 or more days/wk. Will monitor physical activity level at next appointment.
Re-assessment after nutrition intervention	Significant progress toward goal of exercising 30 minutes/day, moderate-intensity activities, 5 or more days/wk. Patient/client reports doing moderate-intensity activities 30 minutes per day, 4 days/week

Suggested references for indicators, measurement techniques, and reference standards are available in the International Dietetics and Nutrition Terminology (IDNT) Reference Manual.

BEHAVIORAL

Edition: 2008

ENERGY INTAKE (FI-1.1)

Definition

Amount of energy intake from all sources (e.g., food, beverages, supplements, and via enteral and parenteral routes)

Monitoring

Changes in these Potential Indicators:
- Total energy intake

Examples of the measurement methods or data sources for these outcome indicators
Food intake records, 24-hour recall, 3-5 day food diary, food frequency questionnaire, caretaker intake records, menu analysis, intake and output records

Typically used to measure the outcomes for the following domains of nutrition interventions
Food and/or nutrient delivery, nutrition education, nutrition counseling, coordination of nutrition care

Typically used to monitor and evaluate change in the following nutrition diagnosis
Inadequate energy intake, excessive energy intake, evident protein-calorie malnutrition, inadequate protein-energy intake, underweight, involuntary weight loss, overweight/obesity, involuntary weight gain, swallowing difficulty, breastfeeding difficulty, altered GI function, limited adherence to nutrition-related recommendations

Evaluation

Criteria for evaluation
Comparison to Goal or Reference Standard:
1. Goal (tailored to individual's needs)
OR
2. Reference standard

ENERGY INTAKE (FI-1.1)

Patient/Client Example(s)

Example(s) of one or two of the Nutrition Care Indicators for this outcome (*includes sample initial and re-assessment documentation for one of the indicators*)

Indicator(s) selected

Total energy intake

Criteria for evaluation

Comparison to Goal or Reference Standard:

1. Goal: Food diary indicates patient/client consumes 2600 kcal/day. Patient/client to target an intake of 1800 kcal/day.

   OR

2. Reference standard: Patient/client's I & O indicates patient/client's intake at 2000 kcal, 75% of goal based on an estimated energy requirement of 2665 kcal/day.

Sample monitoring and evaluation documentation

Initial encounter with patient/client	Based on patient/client food diary, patient/client consuming approximately 2600 kcal/day, 144% of recommended level of 1800 kcals. Will evaluate calorie intake at next encounter in two weeks.
Re-assessment after nutrition intervention	Significant progress toward recommended kcal intake. Based upon food diary, patient/client decreased calorie consumption to 2100 kcal, 117% recommended level. Will assess kcal intake in four weeks.

Suggested references for indicators, measurement techniques, and reference standards are available in the International Dietetics and Nutrition Terminology (IDNT) Reference Manual.

Edition: 2008

FOOD/ NUTRIENT

FLUID/BEVERAGE INTAKE (FI-2.1)

Definition
Amount and type of fluid/beverage intake from all sources (e.g., beverages, supplements, and via enteral and parenteral routes)

Monitoring
Changes in these Potential Indicators:
- Oral fluid amounts
  - o Water
  - o Coffee and tea
  - o Juice
  - o Milk
  - o Soda (regular or artificial sweetened)
- Food-derived fluids
- IV fluids
- Liquid meal replacement

Examples of the measurement methods or data sources for these outcome indicators
Food intake records, 24-hour recall, food frequency questionnaire, menu analysis, intake and output data, number of urinations per day

Typically used to measure the outcomes for the following domains of nutrition interventions
Food and/or nutrient delivery, nutrition education, nutrition counseling, coordination of nutrition care

Typically used to monitor and evaluate change in the following nutrition diagnosis
Excessive or inadequate oral food/beverage intake, food-medication interaction, underweight, overweight/obesity, disordered eating pattern, undesirable food choices, limited adherence to nutrition related recommendations, inability or lack of desire to manage self-care, swallowing difficulty, breastfeeding difficulty, altered GI function

FOOD/
NUTRIENT

FLUID/BEVERAGE INTAKE (FI-2.1)

Evaluation

Criteria for evaluation

Comparison to Goal or Reference Standard:
1. Goal (tailored to patient/client's needs)
OR
2. Reference standard

Patient/Client Example(s)

Example(s) of one or two of the Nutrition Care Indicators for this outcome (*includes sample initial and re-assessment documentation for one of the indicators*)

Indicator(s) selected

Oral fluid amounts

Criteria for evaluation

Comparison to Goal or Reference Standard:
1. Goal: Patient /client currently drinks 12 oz of water per day and has a goal of consuming 64 oz of water per day.
OR
2. Reference standard: Patient/client's intake of 1000 mL of free water (0.8 mL/ kcal) is below the 1mL/kcal guideline.

Sample monitoring and evaluation documentation

Initial encounter with patient/ client	Based on patient/client food diary, patient/client consuming approximately 1000 mL water per day. Will monitor water intake at next encounter.
Re-assessment after nutrition intervention	Significant progress toward recommended water intake. Based upon fluid intake records, patient/client increased consumption of water from 1000 mL to 2600 mL per day.

Suggested references for indicators, measurement techniques, and reference standards are available in the International Dietetics and Nutrition Terminology (IDNT) Reference Manual.

FOOD/ NUTRIENT

Edition: 2008

FOOD INTAKE (FI-2.2)

Definition
Amount, type and quality of food consumed orally

Monitoring
Changes in these Potential Indicators:
- Food variety
- Number of food group servings
  - o Grains
  - o Fruits
  - o Vegetables
  - o Milk/Dairy Foods
  - o Meat/Protein Substitutes (beans, eggs. peanut butter, tofu)
- Healthy Eating Index (HEI)
- Children's Diet Quality Index (C-DQI)
- Revised Children's Diet Quality Index (RC-DQI)

Examples of the measurement methods or data sources for these outcome indicators
Food intake records, 24-hour recall, food frequency questionnaire, menu analysis, MyPyramid Tracker, Healthy Eating Index, C-DQI, RC-DQI

Typically used to measure the outcomes for the following domains of nutrition interventions
Food and/or nutrient delivery, nutrition education, nutrition counseling, coordination of nutrition care

Typically used to monitor and evaluate change in the following nutrition diagnosis
Excessive or inadequate oral food/beverage intake, food-medication interaction, underweight, overweight/obesity, disordered eating pattern, undesirable food choices, limited adherence to nutrition related recommendations, inability or lack of desire to manage self-care.

FOOD INTAKE (FI-2.2)

Evaluation

Criteria for evaluation
Comparison to Goal or Reference Standard:
1. Goal (tailored to patient/client needs)
OR
2. Reference standard

Patient/Client Example(s)
Example(s) of one or two of the Nutrition Care Indicators for this outcome (*includes sample initial and re-assessment documentation for one of the indicators*)

Indicator(s) selected
Number of food group servings

Criteria for evaluation
Comparison to Goal or Reference Standard:
1. Goal: Patient/client currently eats approximately 1-2 fruit and vegetable servings per day. Goal is to increase fruit and vegetable intake to 5 servings per day.
OR
2. Reference standard: Patient/client's current intake of 1-2 servings of fruit and vegetable servings per day is below the 2005 *Dietary Guidelines for Americans* recommendation of 2 cups of fruit and 2 ½ cups of vegetables per day.

Sample monitoring and evaluation documentation

Initial encounter with patient/ client	Based on patient/client recall, patient/client consuming approximately 1-2 servings of fruits and vegetables per day. Will monitor fruit and vegetable intake at next encounter.
Re-assessment after nutrition intervention	Significant progress toward goal of 5 servings of fruit and vegetables per day. Based upon food records, patient/client increased consumption of fruits and vegetables from approximately 1 to 4 servings per day.

Suggested references for indicators, measurement techniques, and reference standards are available in the International Dietetics and Nutrition Terminology (IDNT) Reference Manual.

FOOD/
NUTRIENT

Edition: 2008

ENTERAL AND PARENTERAL NUTRITION INTAKE (FI-3.1)

Definition
Amount or type of enteral and/or parenteral nutrition

Monitoring
Changes in these Potential Indicators:
- Access
- Formula/solution
- Discontinuation
- Initiation
- Rate/schedule

Examples of the measurement methods or data sources for these outcome indicators
Patient/client report/recall, patient/client record, home evaluation, pharmacy report

Typically used to measure the outcomes for the following domains of nutrition interventions
Food and/or nutrient delivery, coordination of nutrition care

Typically used to monitor and evaluate change in the following nutrition diagnoses
Inadequate or excess intake of enteral or parenteral nutrition

Evaluation

Criteria for evaluation
Comparison to Goal or Reference Standard:
1. Goal (tailored to patient/client needs)
   OR
2. Reference standard

ENTERAL AND PARENTERAL NUTRITION INTAKE (FI-3.1)

Patient/Client Example(s)

Example(s) of one or two of the Nutrition Care Indicators for this outcome (*includes sample initial and re-assessment documentation for one of the indicators*)

Indicator(s) selected
Rate/schedule

Criteria for evaluation
Comparison to Goal or Reference Standard:

1. Goal: Patient/client's enteral nutrition is at a rate of 50 mL per hour of 1 calorie per mL formula compared to the nutrition prescription of 80 mL/hour to meet estimated nutrition needs.

   OR

2. Reference standard: There is no reference standard for this outcome because the provision of EN/PN is individualized.

Sample monitoring and evaluation documentation

Initial encounter with patient/ client	Monitor enteral nutrition initiation and rate advancement.
Re-assessment after nutrition intervention	Enteral nutrition at 70 mL per hour. Significant progress toward nutrition prescription of 1 calorie per mL formula at 80 mL per hour.

Suggested references for indicators, measurement techniques, and reference standards are available in the International Dietetics and Nutrition Terminology (IDNT) Reference Manual.

FOOD/
NUTRIENT

Edition: 2008

CHANGE IN ALCOHOL INTAKE (FI-4.1)

Definition
Alteration in alcohol consumption and pattern

Monitoring
Changes in these Potential Indicators:
- Drink size/volume
- Frequency

Examples of the measurement methods or data sources for these outcome indicators
Patient/client report/recall, three item questionnaire, self-monitoring log, 24 hour recall

Typically used to measure the outcomes for the following domains of nutrition interventions
Nutrition education, nutrition counseling

Typically used to monitor and evaluate change in the following nutrition diagnoses
Excess intake of alcohol; excess or inadequate intake of energy; altered nutrition-related laboratory values; impaired nutrient utilization; overweight/obesity

Evaluation

Criteria for evaluation
Comparison to Goal or Reference Standard:
    1. Goal (tailored to patient/client needs)
    OR
    2. Reference standard

FOOD/
NUTRIENT

CHANGE IN ALCOHOL INTAKE (FI-4.1)

Patient/Client Example(s)

Example(s) of one or two of the Nutrition Care Indicators for this outcome (*includes sample initial and re-assessment documentation for one of the indicators*)

Indicator(s) selected

• Drink size/volume
• Frequency

Criteria for evaluation

Comparison to Goal or Reference Standard:

1. Goal: Patient/client's intake of one 5-ounce glass of wine 2-3 times per week is significantly above and noncompliant with the goal to abstain from alcohol during pregnancy.

OR

2. Reference standard: Patient/client's intake of three to four 5-ounce glasses of wine per day is significantly above* the reference standard of one 5-ounce glass of wine per day for women.

Sample monitoring and evaluation documentation

Initial encounter with patient/ client	Based upon recall, patient/client consuming three to four 5-ounce glasses of wine per day. Will monitor change in alcohol intake at next encounter.
Re-assessment after nutrition intervention	Significant progress toward reference standard one 5-ounce glass of wine per day. Based upon 3-day record, patient/client consuming 8 ounces of wine total over the 3-day period.

Suggested references for indicators, measurement techniques, and reference standards are available in the International Dietetics and Nutrition Terminology (IDNT) Reference Manual.

*Could be specified as "above," "below," or a "percent of" the reference value.

BIOACTIVE SUBSTANCE INTAKE (FI-4.2)

Definition

Amount and type of bioactive substances consumed

NOTE: Working definition of bioactive substances—physiologically active components of foods that may offer health benefits beyond traditional macro- or micronutrient requirements. Note: There is no scientific consensus about a definition for bioactive substances/components.

Monitoring

Changes in these Potential Indicators:
- Plant sterol and stanol esters
- Soy protein
- Psyllium and β-glucan

Examples of the measurement methods or data sources for these outcome indicators

Patient/client report/recall, self-monitoring log

Typically used to measure the outcomes for the following domains of nutrition interventions

Nutrition education, nutrition counseling

Typically used to monitor and evaluate change in the following nutrition diagnoses

Inadequate or excess intake of bioactive substances, food-medication interaction

Evaluation

Criteria for evaluation

Comparison to Goal or Reference Standard:
1. Goal (tailored to patient/client needs)
   OR
2. Reference standard

BIOACTIVE SUBSTANCE INTAKE (FI-4.2)

Patient/Client Example(s)

Example(s) of one or two of the Nutrition Care Indicators for this outcome (*includes sample initial and re-assessment documentation for one of the indicators*)

Indicator(s) selected

Plant sterol and stanol esters

Criteria for evaluation

Comparison to Goal or Reference Standard:
1. Goal: The patient/client does not consume plant sterol or stanol esters compared to the goal intake of 2-3 grams per day.
   OR
2. Reference standard: No validated standard exists.

Sample monitoring and evaluation documentation

Initial encounter with patient/ client	Based upon recall, patient/client consuming approximately 0 grams of stanol/sterol ester per day. Will monitor change in stanol/sterol ester intake at next encounter.
Re-assessment after nutrition intervention	No progress toward the goal of 2-3 g/day of stanol/sterol ester. Based upon 3-day diet record, patient/client still consuming 0 grams stanol/sterol ester per day.

Suggested references for indicators, measurement techniques, and reference standards are available in the International Dietetics and Nutrition Terminology (IDNT) Reference Manual.

FOOD/
NUTRIENT

CAFFEINE INTAKE (FI-4.3)

Definition

Amount of caffeine intake from all sources (e.g., food, beverages, supplements, and via enteral and parenteral routes)

Monitoring

Changes in these Potential Indicators:

- Total caffeine intake
  (e.g., naturally occurring caffeine in leaves, seeds, fruits of plants and sources with added caffeine such as, water/beverages, medications)

Examples of the measurement methods or data sources for these outcome indicators
Patient/client report/recall, self-monitoring log

Typically used to measure the outcomes for the following domains of nutrition interventions
Nutrition education, nutrition counseling

Typically used to monitor and evaluate change in the following nutrition diagnoses
Food- and nutrition-related knowledge deficit

Evaluation

Criteria for evaluation
Comparison to Goal or Reference Standard:
1. Goal (tailored to patient/client needs)
   OR
2. Reference standard

FOOD/
NUTRIENT

CAFFEINE INTAKE (FI-4.3)

Patient/Client Example(s)

Example(s) of one or two of the Nutrition Care Indicators for this outcome (*includes sample initial and re-assessment documentation for one of the indicators*)

Indicator(s) selected
Total caffeine intake

Criteria for evaluation
Comparison to Goal or Reference Standard:

1. Goal: The patient/client's intake is 600 mg of caffeine per day, which is above the goal of < 300 mg caffeine per day.

   OR

2. Reference standard: The patient/client's intake is approximately 600 mg of caffeine per day which is 150%* of the reference standard of 400 mg caffeine per day.

Sample monitoring and evaluation documentation

Initial encounter with patient/ client	Based upon recall, patient/client consuming approximately 600 mg caffeine per day. Will monitor change in caffeine intake at next encounter.
Re-assessment after nutrition intervention	No progress toward the reference standard of 400 mg for caffeine. Based upon 3-day diet record, patient/client still consuming 600 mg caffeine per day.

Suggested references for indicators, measurement techniques, and reference standards are available in the International Dietetics and Nutrition Terminology (IDNT) Reference Manual.

*Could be specified as "above," "below," or a "percent of" the reference value.

FOOD/
NUTRIENT

FAT AND CHOLESTEROL INTAKE (FI-5.1)

Definition
Fat and cholesterol consumption from all sources, e.g., food, beverages, supplements, and via enteral and parenteral routes

Monitoring
Changes in these Potential Indicators:
- Total fat (grams or % of calories)
- Saturated fat (grams or % of calories)
- *Trans* fatty acids (grams or % of calories)
- Polyunsaturated fat (grams or % of calories)
- Monounsaturated fat (grams or % of calories)
- Omega-3 fatty acids
    - o Marine-derived
    - o Plant-derived
        - Alpha-linolenic acid (amount or % of calories)
- Dietary cholesterol

NOTE: Plant sterol and stanol esters can be found on the Bioactive Substance Intake Reference Sheet.

Examples of the measurement methods or data sources for these outcome indicators
Food intake records, 24-hour recall, food frequency questionnaires, menu analysis, fat and cholesterol targeted questionnaires and monitoring devices

Typically used to measure the outcomes for the following domains of nutrition interventions
Food and/or nutrient delivery, nutrition education, nutrition counseling

Typically used to monitor and evaluate change in the following nutrition diagnosis
Inadequate and excessive fat intake, inappropriate intake of food fats, overweight/ obesity, altered nutrition-related lab values, altered food and nutrition-related knowledge deficit

FAT AND CHOLESTEROL INTAKE (FI-5.1)

Evaluation

Criteria for evaluation

Comparison to Goal or Reference Standard:
1. Goal (tailored to patient/client's needs)
   OR
2. Reference standard

Patient/Client Example(s)

Example(s) of one or two of the Nutrition Care Indicators for this outcome (*includes sample initial and re-assessment documentation for one of the indicators*)

Indicator(s) selected

- Total fat (grams or % of calories)
- Dietary cholesterol

Criteria for evaluation

Comparison to Goal or Reference Standard:
1. Goal: Patient/client currently consumes 50% of calories from fat. Goal is to decrease fat intake to 40% of calories.
   OR
2. Reference standard: Patient/client's intake of 350 mg of cholesterol per day is 175% of the Adult Treatment Panel III guidelines of less than 200 mg of dietary cholesterol per day.

Sample monitoring and evaluation documentation

Initial encounter with patient/ client	Based upon a three-day food diary, patient/client is consuming approximately 50% of calories from fat. Patient/ client goal is to reduce total fat intake to 40% of calories. Will monitor fat and calorie intake at next appointment.
Re-assessment after nutrition intervention	Significant progress toward the goal intake of 40% calories from fat. Based on a three-day food diary patient/client's total fat intake decreased from approximately 50% to 44% calories from fat/day. Will continue to monitor progress at next encounter in 6 weeks.

Suggested references for indicators, measurement techniques, and reference standards are available in the International Dietetics and Nutrition Terminology (IDNT) Reference Manual.

FOOD/ NUTRIENT

Edition: 2008

PROTEIN INTAKE (FI-5.2)

Definition
Protein intake from all sources (e.g., food, beverages, supplements, and via enteral and parenteral routes)

Monitoring
Changes in these Potential Indicators:
- Total protein
- High biological value protein
- Casein
- Whey
- Soy protein*
- Amino acids
- Essential amino acids

*Soy protein can be found on the Bioactive Substance Intake Reference Sheet.

Examples of the measurement methods or data sources for these outcome indicators
Food intake records, 24-hour recall, food frequency questionnaires, menu analysis, protein intake collection tools

Typically used to measure the outcomes for the following domains of nutrition interventions
Food and/or nutrient delivery, nutrition education, nutrition counseling, coordination of nutrition care

Typically used to monitor and evaluate change in the following nutrition diagnosis
Inadequate and excessive protein intake, inappropriate intake of amino acids, evident protein-energy malnutrition, inadequate protein-energy intake, swallowing difficulty, breastfeeding difficulty, altered GI function, limited adherence to nutrition-related recommendations

Evaluation

Criteria for evaluation
Comparison to Goal or Reference Standard:
1. Goal (tailored to patient/client's needs)
   OR
2. Reference standard

FOOD/
NUTRIENT

PROTEIN INTAKE (FI-5.2)

Patient/Client Example(s)

Example(s) of one or two of the Nutrition Care Indicators for this outcome (*includes sample initial and re-assessment documentation for one of the indicators*)

Indicator(s) selected
Total protein

Criteria for evaluation
Comparison to Goal or Reference Standard:

1. Goal: Patient/client's current intake of 25 g protein per day is below the recommended level of 55–65 g per day.

OR

2. Reference standard: (Used when patient goal is based on the population standard) Patient/client's intake of 12 g protein/day is less then the DRI of 53 g/day (0.8 g/kg BW). Patient/client's goal is to increase protein intake to approximately 55 g/day.

Sample monitoring and evaluation documentation

Initial encounter with patient/ client	Enteral feeding currently providing 25 g protein/day, well below the recommended level of 55–65 g/day (1-1.2 g/kg BW). Will continue to monitor protein intake daily.
Re-assessment after nutrition intervention	Some progress toward goal intake of 55–65 g protein/day. Current intake approximately 30 g protein/day, 25 g protein below desired level. Will continue to monitor protein intake daily.

Suggested references for indicators, measurement techniques, and reference standards are available in the International Dietetics and Nutrition Terminology (IDNT) Reference Manual.

FOOD/
NUTRIENT

Edition: 2008

CARBOHYDRATE INTAKE (FI-5.3)

Definition

Carbohydrate consumption from all sources, (e.g., food, beverages, supplements, and via enteral and parenteral routes)

Monitoring

Changes in these Potential Indicators:

- Total carbohydrate
- Sugar
- Starch
- Glycemic index
- Glycemic load

NOTE: Fiber intake is listed on the Fiber Intake Reference Sheet.

Examples of the measurement methods or data sources for these outcome indicators

Food intake records, 24-hour recall, food frequency questionnaires, menu analysis, carbohydrate counting tools

Typically used to measure the outcomes for the following domains of nutrition interventions

Food and/or nutrient delivery, nutrition education, nutrition counseling, coordination of nutrition care

Typically used to monitor and evaluate change in the following nutrition diagnosis

Inadequate and excessive carbohydrate intake, inappropriate intake of types of carbohydrate, inconsistent carbohydrate intake

Evaluation

Criteria for evaluation

Comparison to Goal or Reference Standard:

1. Goal (tailored to patient/client's needs)

OR

2. Reference standard

CARBOHYDRATE INTAKE (FI-5.3)

Patient/Client Example(s)

Example(s) of one or two of the Nutrition Care Indicators for this outcome (*includes sample initial and re-assessment documentation for one of the indicators*)

Indicator(s) selected

Total carbohydrate (distribution by meal)

Criteria for evaluation

Comparison to Goal or Reference Standard:

1. Goal: Patient/client's current carbohydrate intake in the morning is inconsistent. Patient/client will consume approximately 30 g carbohydrate at breakfast.

OR

2. Reference standard: No validated standard exists.

Sample monitoring and evaluation documentation

Initial encounter with patient/ client	Based upon carbohydrate counting tools, patient/client consumes 30 g carbohydrate at breakfast 2 days/week. Goal is to consume 30 g carbohydrate 6 days per week.
Re-assessment after nutrition intervention	Based upon carbohydrate counting tools, patient/client consumed 30 g carbohydrate at breakfast 2 days/week. No progress made in this indicator. Will monitor carbohydrate intake at breakfast at next encounter.

Suggested references for indicators, measurement techniques, and reference standards are available in the International Dietetics and Nutrition Terminology (IDNT) Reference Manual.

FOOD/ NUTRIENT

Edition: 2008

FIBER INTAKE (FI-5.4)

Definition

Amount and/or type of indigested carbohydrate from all sources (e.g., food, beverages, supplements, and via enteral routes)

Monitoring

Changes in these Potential Indicators:

- Total Fiber
- Soluble Fiber
- Insoluble Fiber
    - o   Fructooligosaccharides

NOTE: Psyllium and β-glucan can be found on the Bioactive Substance Intake Reference Sheet

Examples of the measurement methods or data sources for these outcome indicators

Food intake records, 24-hour recall, food frequency questionnaires, menu analysis, fiber counting tools

Typically used to measure the outcomes for the following domains of nutrition interventions

Food and/or nutrient delivery, nutrition education, nutrition counseling, coordination of nutrition care

Typically used to monitor and evaluate change in the following nutrition diagnosis

Inadequate and excessive fiber intake, altered GI function

Evaluation

Criteria for evaluation

Comparison to Goal or Reference Standard:

1. Goal (tailored to patient/client's needs)

OR

2. Reference standard

FIBER INTAKE (FI-5.4)

Patient/Client Example(s)

Example(s) of one or two of the Nutrition Care Indicators for this outcome (*includes sample initial and re-assessment documentation for one of the indicators*)

Indicator(s) selected
Total fiber

Criteria for evaluation
Comparison to Goal or Reference Standard:
1. Goal: Patient/client with current fiber intake of 15 g per day. Goal is to increase fiber intake to approximately 25 g per day.

OR

2. Reference standard: Patient/client's current intake of 15 g of dietary fiber per day is below the DRI of 25 g/day for a 40-year-old woman.

Sample monitoring and evaluation documentation

Initial encounter with patient/ client	Based upon patient/client's food diary, patient/client is consuming approximately 15 g of fiber/day. Will monitor fiber intake at next encounter in three weeks.
Re-assessment after nutrition intervention	Goal achieved. Patient/client's intake of 27 g fiber exceeded goal intake of 25 g/day. Will continue to monitor to ensure success is sustained.

Suggested references for indicators, measurement techniques, and reference standards are available in the International Dietetics and Nutrition Terminology (IDNT) Reference Manual.

FOOD/ NUTRIENT

VITAMIN INTAKE (FI-6.1)

Definition
Vitamin intake from all sources (e.g., food, beverages, supplements, and via enteral and parenteral routes)

Monitoring
Changes in these Potential Indicators:
- Vitamin A
- Vitamin C
- Vitamin D
- Vitamin E
- Vitamin K
- Thiamin
- Riboflavin
- Niacin
- Vitamin B6
- Folate
- Vitamin B12
- Pantothenic acid
- Biotin
- Choline

Examples of the measurement methods or data sources for these outcome indicators
Patient/client report or recall, food frequency, home evaluation, supplement use questionnaire

Typically used to measure the outcomes for the following domains of nutrition interventions
Food and/or nutrient delivery, nutrition education, nutrition counseling, coordination of nutrition care

Typically used to monitor and evaluate change in the following nutrition diagnoses
Excess or inadequate intake of vitamins, parenteral, or enteral nutrition

Evaluation

Criteria for evaluation
Comparison to Goal or Reference Standard:
1. Nutrition prescription or goal (tailored to patient/client needs)
   OR
2. Reference standard

VITAMIN INTAKE (FI-6.1)

Patient/Client Example(s)

Example(s) of one or two of the Nutrition Care Indicators for this outcome (*includes sample initial and re-assessment documentation for one of the indicators*)

Indicator(s) selected
Vitamin D

Criteria for evaluation
Comparison to Goal or Reference Standard:
1. Nutrition prescription or goal: Use if patient/client's nutrition prescription/ goal is different from the reference standard.
OR
2. Reference standard: The patient/client's intake of 2 μg of vitamin D is 20%* of the adequate intake (AI) for men age 51 and older.

Sample monitoring and evaluation documentation

Initial encounter with patient/ client	Based upon recall, patient/client consuming approximately 20% of the adequate intake (AI) for vitamin D per day. Will monitor vitamin D intake at next encounter.
Re-assessment after nutrition intervention	Significant progress toward the adequate intake of 10 μg for vitamin D. Based upon 3-day diet record, patient/client has increased consumption of vitamin D from 50% to 75% of the adequate intake per day.

Suggested references for indicators, measurement techniques, and reference standards are available in the International Dietetics and Nutrition Terminology (IDNT) Reference Manual.

*Could be specified as "above," "below," or a "percent of" the reference value.

FOOD/
NUTRIENT

Edition: 2008

MINERAL/ELEMENT INTAKE (FI-6.2)

Definition
Mineral/element intake from all sources (e.g., food, beverages, supplements, and via enteral and parenteral routes)

Monitoring
Changes in these Potential Indicators:
- Calcium
- Copper
- Fluoride
- Iodine
- Iron
- Magnesium
- Phosphorus
- Selenium
- Zinc
- Potassium
- Sodium
- Chloride
- Chromium

Examples of the measurement methods or data sources for these outcome indicators
Patient/client report or recall, food frequency, home evaluation, home care or pharmacy report, supplement use questionnaire

Typically used to measure the outcomes for the following domains of nutrition interventions
Food and/or nutrient delivery, nutrition education, nutrition counseling, coordination of nutrition care

Typically used to monitor and evaluate change in the following nutrition diagnoses
Excess or inadequate intake of minerals

Evaluation

Criteria for evaluation
Comparison to Goal or Reference Standard:
1. Nutrition prescription or goal (tailored to individual's needs)
OR
2. Reference standard

MINERAL/ELEMENT INTAKE (FI-6.2)

Patient/Client Example(s)

Example(s) of one or two of the Nutrition Care Indicators for this outcome (*includes sample initial and re-assessment documentation for one of the indicators*)

Indicator(s) selected
- Sodium
- Calcium

Criteria for evaluation

Comparison to Goal or Reference Standard:

1. Nutrition prescription or goal: The patient/client's intake of sodium is approximately 6000 mg per day compared to the nutrition prescription of 4000 mg per day.

OR

2. Reference standard: The patient/client's intake of calcium is 500 mg per day which is 50%* of the Adequate Intake (AI) for women 31-50 years of age.

Sample monitoring and evaluation documentation

Initial encounter with patient/ client	Based upon recall, patient/client consuming approximately 50% of the adequate intake for calcium per day. Will monitor calcium intake at next encounter.
Re-assessment after nutrition intervention	Significant progress toward the adequate intake of 1000 mg of calcium per day. Based upon 3-day diet record, patient/ client has increased consumption from 50% to 75% of the adequate daily intake for calcium.

Suggested references for indicators, measurement techniques, and reference standards are available in the International Dietetics and Nutrition Terminology (IDNT) Reference Manual.

*Could be specified as "above," "below," or a "percent of" the reference value.

 Edition: 2008

BODY COMPOSITION/GROWTH (S-1.1)

Definition
The body's fat, muscle, and bone tissue, including growth

Monitoring
Changes in these Potential Indicators:
- Body mass index
- Ideal body weight (IBW) or usual body weight (UBW) percentage
- Growth pattern (head circumference, length/height, weight for length/stature, BMI percentile/age (*Also see Weight change below*)
- Weight, weight change (e.g., % change for adults, weight gain [e.g., g/day for neonates])
- Lean body mass, fat free mass
- Mid-arm muscle circumference
- Body fat percentage
- Triceps skin fold
- Waist circumference
- Waist hip ratio
- Bone age
- Bone mineral density

Examples of the measurement methods or data sources for these outcome indicators
Direct measurement, patient/client report, medical record

Typically used to measure the outcomes for the following domains of nutrition interventions
Food and nutrient delivery, nutrition education, nutrition counseling

Typically used to monitor and evaluate change in the following nutrition diagnoses
Excess or inadequate intake of energy, fat, protein, carbohydrate, alcohol, and/or mineral intake; underweight, overweight, physical inactivity, excessive exercise

BODY COMPOSITION/GROWTH (S-1.1)

Evaluation

Criteria for evaluation

Comparison to Goal or Reference Standard:

1. Goal (tailored to patient/client's needs)
   OR
2. Reference standard

Patient/Client Example(s)

Example(s) of one or two of the Nutrition Care Indicators for this outcome (*includes sample initial and re-assessment documentation for one of the indicators*)

Indicator(s) selected

- Weight gain/day
- BMI percentile/age

Criteria for evaluation

Comparison to Goal or Reference Standard:

1. Goal: The infant is only gaining, on average, 10 grams per day compared with a goal weight gain of 20–30 grams per day.
   OR
2. Reference standard: Child's (> age 3 years) BMI percentile/age per growth curves has crossed 2 percentiles from 50% to 10% in last 6 months.

Sample monitoring and evaluation documentation

Initial encounter with patient/ client	Child's BMI percentile/age per growth curves has crossed 2 percentiles from 50% to 10% in last 6 months. Will monitor BMI percentile/age at next encounter.
Re-assessment after nutrition intervention	Child's BMI percentile/age per growth curves is unchanged from baseline measure.

Suggested references for indicators, measurement techniques, and reference standards are available in the International Dietetics and Nutrition Terminology (IDNT) Reference Manual.

SIGN/ SYMPTOM

Edition: 2008

ACID-BASE BALANCE (S-2.1)

Definition
Degree of acidity and alkalinity in the blood as measured by the systemic arterial pH

Monitoring
Changes in these Potential Indicators:
- pH, serum
- Bicarbonate (HCO_3)
- Partial pressure of carbon dioxide in arterial blood ($PaCO_2$)

NOTE: Sodium and Chloride can be found on the Electrolyte and Renal Profile reference sheet.

Examples of the measurement methods or data sources for these outcome indicators
Biochemical measurement, laboratory report

Typically used to measure the outcomes for the following domains of nutrition interventions
Food and/or nutrient delivery, coordination of nutrition care

Typically used to monitor and evaluate change in the following nutrition diagnoses
Excess intake of parenteral or enteral nutrition

Evaluation

Criteria for evaluation
Comparison to Goal or Reference Standard:
1. Goal (tailored to patient/client's needs)
OR
2. Reference standard

SIGN/
SYMPTOM

ACID-BASE BALANCE (S-2.1)

Patient/Client Example(s)

Example(s) of one or two of the Nutrition Care Indicators for this outcome (*includes sample initial and re-assessment documentation for one of the indicators*)

Indicator(s) selected
pH

Criteria for evaluation
Comparison to Goal or Reference Standard:
1. Goal: Not generally used for this outcome.
OR
2. Reference standard: The patient/client pH is 7.48 which is above* the reference standard (7.35-7.45).

Sample monitoring and evaluation documentation

Initial encounter with patient/ client	Patient/client's pH is 7.48. Will monitor change in pH at next blood gas.
Re-assessment after nutrition intervention	Significant progress toward reference standard. Patient/ client's pH is 7.45.

Suggested references for indicators, measurement techniques, and reference standards are available in the International Dietetics and Nutrition Terminology (IDNT) Reference Manual.

*Could be specified as "above," "below," or a "percent of" the reference value.

SIGN/
SYMPTOM

ELECTROLYTE AND RENAL PROFILE (S-2.2)

Definition
Laboratory measures associated with electrolyte balance and kidney function

Monitoring
Changes in these Potential Indicators:
- BUN
- Creatinine
- BUN:creatinine ratio
- Glomerular filtration rate
- Sodium
- Chloride
- Potassium
- Magnesium
- Calcium
- Calcium, ionized
- Phosphorus
- Serum osmolality
- Parathyroid hormone

NOTE: Bicarbonate can be found on the Acid Base Balance reference sheet.

Examples of the measurement methods or data sources for these outcome indicators
Biochemical measurement, laboratory report

Typically used to measure the outcomes for the following domains of nutrition interventions
Food and/or nutrient delivery, coordination of nutrition care

Typically used to monitor and evaluate change in the following nutrition diagnoses
Excess or inadequate intake of protein or minerals

ELECTROLYTE AND RENAL PROFILE (S-2.2)

Evaluation

Criteria for evaluation
Comparison to Goal or Reference Standard:
1. Goal (tailored to patient/client's needs)
OR
2. Reference standard

Patient/Client Example(s)
Example(s) of one or two of the Nutrition Care Indicators for this outcome (*includes sample initial and re-assessment documentation for one of the indicators*)

Indicator(s) selected
Potassium

Criteria for evaluation
Comparison to Goal or Reference Standard:
1. Goal: Not generally used for this outcome.
OR
2. Reference standard: The patient/client's potassium is 2.9 mEq/L which is below* the reference standard (3.5-5.0 mEq/L).

Sample monitoring and evaluation documentation

Initial encounter with patient/ client	Patient/client's serum potassium is 2.9 mEq/L. Will monitor change in potassium at next encounter.
Re-assessment after nutrition intervention	Regression from reference standard. Patient/client's potassium is 2.7 mEq/L.

Suggested references for indicators, measurement techniques, and reference standards are available in the International Dietetics and Nutrition Terminology (IDNT) Reference Manual.

*Could be specified as "above," "below," or a "percent of" the reference value.

SIGN/
SYMPTOM

Edition: 2008

ESSENTIAL FATTY ACID PROFILE (S-2.3)

Definition
Laboratory measures of essential fatty acids

Monitoring
Changes in these Potential Indicators:
- Triene:Tetraene ratio

Examples of the measurement methods or data sources for these outcome indicators
Biochemical measurement, laboratory report/record

Typically used to measure the outcomes for the following domains of nutrition interventions
Food and/or nutrient delivery, coordination of nutrition care

Typically used to monitor and evaluate change in the following nutrition diagnoses
Inadequate intake of fat, parenteral nutrition; inappropriate intake of parenteral nutrition; altered nutrition-related laboratory values; impaired nutrient utilization

Evaluation

Criteria for evaluation
Comparison to Goal or Reference Standard:
1. Goal (tailored to patient/client's needs)
   OR
2. Reference standard

ESSENTIAL FATTY ACID PROFILE (S-2.3)

Patient/Client Example(s)

Example(s) of one or two of the Nutrition Care Indicators for this outcome (*includes sample initial and re-assessment documentation for one of the indicators*)

Indicator(s) selected

Triene:Tetraene ratio

Criteria for evaluation

Comparison to Goal or Reference Standard:
1. Goal: Not generally used for this outcome.
   OR
2. Reference standard: The patient/client's Triene:Tetraene ratio is 0.45, which is above* the reference standard (> 0.2-0.4) indicating essential fatty acid deficiency.

Sample monitoring and evaluation documentation

Initial encounter with patient/ client	Patient/client's Triene:Tetraene ratio is 0.45. Will monitor change in Triene:Tetraene ratio at next encounter.
Re-assessment after nutrition intervention	Significant progress toward reference standard. Patient/ client's Triene:Tetraene ratio is 0.1.

Suggested references for indicators, measurement techniques, and reference standards are available in the International Dietetics and Nutrition Terminology (IDNT) Reference Manual.

*Could be specified as "above," "below," or a "percent of" the reference value.

GASTROINTESTINAL PROFILE (S-2.4)

Definition
Laboratory measures associated with function of the gastrointestinal tract and related organs

Monitoring
Changes in these Potential Indicators:
- Amylase
- Alkaline phophatase
- Alanine aminotransferase (ALT)
- Aspartate aminotransferase (AST)
- Gamma Glutamyl Transferase (GGT)
- Bilirubin, total
- Ammonia, serum
- Prothrombin time (PT)
- Partial thromboplastin time (PTT)
- INR (ratio)
- Fecal fat

Examples of the measurement methods or data sources for these outcome indicators
Biochemical measurement, laboratory report

Typically used to measure the outcomes for the following domains of nutrition interventions
Food and/or nutrient delivery, nutrition education, nutrition counseling

Typically used to monitor and evaluate change in the following nutrition diagnoses
Altered nutrition-related laboratory values, excess intake of protein or fat

GASTROINTESTINAL PROFILE (S-2.4)

Evaluation

Criteria for evaluation
Comparison to Goal or Reference Standard:
1. Goal (tailored to patient/client's needs)
OR
2. Reference standard

Patient/Client Example(s)
Example(s) of one or two of the Nutrition Care Indicators for this outcome (*includes sample initial and re-assessment documentation for one of the indicators*)

Indicator(s) selected
Ammonia, serum

Criteria for evaluation
Comparison to Goal or Reference Standard:
1. Goal: The patient/client's serum ammonia is 105 µg/dL, which is above the goal (< 75 µg/dL) for this patient/client with end-stage liver disease.
OR
2. Reference standard: The patient/client serum ammonia is 85 µg/dL which is above* the reference standard (11-35 µg/dL).

Sample monitoring and evaluation documentation

Initial encounter with patient/ client	Patient/client's serum ammonia is 85 µg/dL. Will monitor change in serum ammonia at next encounter.
Re-assessment after nutrition intervention	Significant progress toward reference standard. Patient/ client's serum ammonia 45 µg/dL.

Suggested references for indicators, measurement techniques, and reference standards are available in the International Dietetics and Nutrition Terminology (IDNT) Reference Manual.

*Could be specified as "above," "below," or a "percent of" the reference value.

SIGN/ SYMPTOM

Edition: 2008

GLUCOSE PROFILE (S-2.5)

Definition
Laboratory measures associated with glycemic control

Monitoring
Changes in these Potential Indicators:
- Glucose, fasting
- Glucose, casual
- HgbA1c
- Preprandial capillary plasma glucose
- Peak postprandial capillary plasma glucose

Examples of the measurement methods or data sources for these outcome indicators
Biochemical measurement, laboratory report

Typically used to measure the outcomes for the following domains of nutrition interventions
Food and/or nutrient delivery, nutrition education, nutrition counseling

Typically used to monitor and evaluate change in the following nutrition diagnoses
Excess or inadequate intake of carbohydrate, energy; inappropriate intake of types of carbohydrates; or inconsistent carbohydrate intake

Evaluation

Criteria for evaluation
Comparison to Goal or Reference Standard:
1. Goal (tailored to patient/client's needs)
   OR
2. Reference standard

GLUCOSE PROFILE (S-2.5)

Patient/Client Example(s)

Example(s) of one or two of the Nutrition Care Indicators for this outcome (*includes sample initial and re-assessment documentation for one of the indicators*)

Indicator(s) selected
HgbA1c

Criteria for evaluation
Comparison to Goal or Reference Standard:
1. Goal: The patient/client's HgbA1c is 7.8%, which is above the reference standard; however, acceptable in this pediatric patient.

OR

2. Reference standard: The patient/client's HgbA1c is 11%, which is above* the reference standard (< 6%).

Sample monitoring and evaluation documentation

Initial encounter with patient/ client	Patient/client's HgbA1c is 9%. Will monitor change in HgbA1c at next encounter.
Re-assessment after nutrition intervention	Regression from reference standard. Patient/client's HgbA1c is 9.5%.

Suggested references for indicators, measurement techniques, and reference standards are available in the International Dietetics and Nutrition Terminology (IDNT) Reference Manual.

*Could be specified as "above," "below," or a "percent of" the reference value.

Edition: 2008

SIGN/
SYMPTOM

LIPID PROFILE (S-2.6)

Definition
Laboratory measures associated with lipid disorders

Monitoring
Changes in these Potential Indicators:
- Cholesterol, serum
- Cholesterol, HDL
- Cholesterol, LDL
- Triglycerides, serum

Examples of the measurement methods or data sources for these outcome indicators
Biochemical measurement, laboratory report, patient/client report

Typically used to measure the outcomes for the following domains of nutrition interventions
Nutrition education, nutrition counseling

Typically used to monitor and evaluate change in the following nutrition diagnoses
Excess or inadequate intake of fat, energy

Evaluation

Criteria for evaluation
Comparison to Goal or Reference Standard:
1. Goal (tailored to patient/client's needs)
   OR
2. Reference standard

LIPID PROFILE (S-2.6)

Patient/Client Example(s)

Example(s) of one or two of the Nutrition Care Indicators for this outcome (*includes sample initial and re-assessment documentation for one of the indicators*)

Indicator(s) selected
LDL-cholesterol

Criteria for evaluation
Comparison to Goal or Reference Standard:
1. Goal: The patient/client's LDL-cholesterol is 200 mg/dL, compared to a goal of < 100 mg/dL. (Note: Although reference standards are generally used for laboratory measures, a goal might be used in a special situation such as this example. The patient/client has a familial hypercholesterolemia where a normal reference standard may not be realistic.)
OR
2. Reference standard: The patient/client's LDL-cholesterol is 159 mg/dL, which is above* the NHLBI recommended level of < 100 mg/dL.

Sample monitoring and evaluation documentation

Initial encounter with patient/ client	The patient/client LDL-cholesterol is 159 mg/dL, compared to the NHLBI recommended level of < 100 mg/dL. Will monitor LDL-cholesterol at next encounter.
Re-assessment after nutrition intervention	Some progress toward goal/reference standard as patient/ client's LDL-cholesterol is 145 mg/dL.

Suggested references for indicators, measurement techniques, and reference standards are available in the International Dietetics and Nutrition Terminology (IDNT) Reference Manual.

*Could be specified as "above," "below," or a "percent of" the reference value.

MINERAL PROFILE (S-2.7)

Definition
Laboratory measures associated with body mineral status

Monitoring
Changes in these Potential Indicators:
- Copper, serum
- Iodine, urinary excretion
- Thyroid stimulating hormone (TSH) (↑ TSH as an indicator of excess iodine supplementation)
- Zinc, plasma

NOTE: Calcium, magnesium, phosphorus, and potassium can be found on the Electrolyte and Renal Profile reference sheet
Serum iron, serum ferritin, and transferrin saturation can be found on the Nutritional Anemia Profile reference sheet

Examples of the measurement methods or data sources for these outcome indicators
Biochemical measurement, laboratory record

Typically used to measure the outcomes for the following domains of nutrition interventions
Food and/or nutrient delivery, nutrition education, nutrition counseling

Typically used to monitor and evaluate change in the following nutrition diagnoses
Excess or inadequate intake of minerals, parenteral nutrition

Evaluation

Criteria for evaluation
Comparison to Goal or Reference Standard:
1. Goal (tailored to patient/client's needs)
   OR
2. Reference standard

MINERAL PROFILE (S-2.7)

Patient/Client Example(s)

Example(s) of one or two of the Nutrition Care Indicators for this outcome (*includes sample initial and re-assessment documentation for one of the indicators*)

Indicator(s) selected
Zinc, plasma

Criteria for evaluation
Comparison to Goal or Reference Standard:
1. Goal: There is no goal generally associated with mineral status.

OR

2. Reference standard: The patient/client's plasma zinc is 40 µg/dL which is below* the reference standard (66-110 µg/dL) for adults.

Sample monitoring and evaluation documentation

Initial encounter with patient/ client	Patient/client's plasma zinc is 40 µg/dL, which is below the reference standard for adults. Will monitor change in plasma zinc at next encounter.
Re-assessment after nutrition intervention	Goal/reference standard achieved as patient/client's plasma zinc is 90 µg/dL.

Suggested references for indicators, measurement techniques, and reference standards are available in the International Dietetics and Nutrition Terminology (IDNT) Reference Manual.

*Could be specified as "above," "below," or a "percent of" the reference value.

SIGN/
SYMPTOM

Edition: 2008

NUTRITIONAL ANEMIA PROFILE (S-2.8)

Definition
Laboratory measures associated with nutritional anemias

Monitoring
Changes in these Potential Indicators:
- Hemoglobin
- Hematocrit
- Mean corpuscular volume (MCV)
- RBC folate
- Red cell distribution width (RDW)
- Serum B12
- Serum methylmalonic acid (MMA)
- Serum folate
- Serum homocysteine
- Serum ferritin
- Serum iron
- Total iron-binding capacity
- Transferrin saturation

Examples of the measurement methods or data sources for these outcome indicators
Biochemical measurement, patient/client laboratory record; national/state/local nutrition monitoring and surveillance data

Typically used to measure the outcomes for the following domains of nutrition interventions
Food and/or nutrient delivery, nutrition education, nutrition counseling

Typically used to monitor and evaluate change in the following nutrition diagnoses
Excess or inadequate intake of vitamins or minerals (e.g., iron, B12, folate); altered nutrition-related laboratory values; impaired nutrient utilization

Evaluation

Criteria for evaluation
Comparison to Goal or Reference Standard:
1. Goal (tailored to patient/client's needs)
   OR
2. Reference standard

NUTRITIONAL ANEMIA PROFILE (S-2.8)

Patient/Client Example(s)

Example(s) of one or two of the Nutrition Care Indicators for this outcome (*includes sample initial and re-assessment documentation for one of the indicators*)

Indicator(s) selected

- Hemoglobin
- Serum ferritin

Criteria for evaluation

Comparison to Goal or Reference Standard:

1. Goal: The patient/client's hemoglobin and hematocrit are below the reference standard for adult males, but are within the goal range for a patient/client receiving hemodialysis.

OR

2. Reference standard: The patient/client's serum ferritin is 8 ng/mL which is below* the reference standard for women.

Sample monitoring and evaluation documentation

Initial encounter with patient/client	Patient/client's serum ferritin is 8 ng/mL which is below the reference standard for adult females. Will monitor change in serum ferritin at next encounter.
Re-assessment after nutrition intervention	Goal/reference standard achieved as patient/client's serum ferritin is 10.9 ng/mL.

Suggested references for indicators, measurement techniques, and reference standards are available in the International Dietetics and Nutrition Terminology (IDNT) Reference Manual.

*Could be specified as "above," "below," or a "percent of" the reference value.

PROTEIN PROFILE (S-2.9)

Definition
Laboratory measures associated with hepatic and circulating proteins

Monitoring
Changes in these Potential Indicators:
- Albumin
- Prealbumin
- Transferrin
- Phenylalanine, plasma
- Tyrosine, plasma

Note: Hepatic proteins may be useful when monitoring nutritional status over time in conjunction with other markers/information about nutritional status (e.g., body weight, weight change, nutrient intake).

Examples of the measurement methods or data sources for these outcome indicators
Biochemical measurement, laboratory report

Typically used to measure the outcomes for the following domains of nutrition interventions
Food and/or nutrient delivery, nutrition education, nutrition counseling, coordination of nutrition care

Typically used to monitor and evaluate change in the following nutrition diagnoses
Increased nutrient needs, evident protein-energy malnutrition, inadequate intake of enteral/parenteral nutrition

Evaluation

Criteria for evaluation
Comparison to Goal or Reference Standard:
1. Goal (tailored to patient/client's needs)
   OR
2. Reference standard

PROTEIN PROFILE (S-2.9)

Patient/Client Example(s)

Example(s) of one or two of the Nutrition Care Indicators for this outcome (*includes sample initial and re-assessment documentation for one of the indicators*)

Indicator(s) selected
Prealbumin

Criteria for evaluation
Comparison to Goal or Reference Standard:
1. Goal: Not generally used for this outcome.

OR

2. Reference standard: The patient/client's prealbumin is 7 mg/dL, which is below* the reference standard (16-40 mg/dL) for adults.

Sample monitoring and evaluation documentation

Initial encounter with patient/ client	Patient/client's prealbumin is 7.0 mg/dL. Will monitor change in pre-albumin at next encounter.
Re-assessment after nutrition intervention	Significant progress toward goal/reference standard as patient/client's serum prealbumin is 13.0 mg/dL.

Suggested references for indicators, measurement techniques, and reference standards are available in the International Dietetics and Nutrition Terminology (IDNT) Reference Manual.

*Could be specified as "above," "below," or a "percent of" the reference value.

SIGN/ SYMPTOM

Edition: 2008

RESPIRATORY QUOTIENT (RQ) (S-2.10)

Definition
Ratio of the volume of carbon dioxide produced to the volume of oxygen consumed, which, under controlled conditions, is a reflection of net substrate utilization in the body

Monitoring
Changes in these Potential Indicators:
- Respiratory quotient (RQ = CO_2 produced/O_2 consumed)

Examples of the measurement methods or data sources for these outcome indicators
Direct measurement, medical record

Typically used to measure the outcomes for the following domains of nutrition interventions
Food and/or nutrient delivery

Typically used to monitor and evaluate change in the following nutrition diagnoses
Excessive or inadequate intake of parenteral/enteral nutrition; inappropriate infusion of enteral/parenteral nutrition

Evaluation

Criteria for evaluation
Comparison to Goal or Reference Standard:
1. Goal (tailored to patient/client's needs)
   OR
2. Reference standard

RESPIRATORY QUOTIENT (RQ) (S-2.10)

Patient/Client Example(s)

Example(s) of one or two of the Nutrition Care Indicators for this outcome (*includes sample initial and re-assessment documentation for one of the indicators*)

Indicator(s) selected

RQ

Criteria for evaluation

Comparison to Goal or Reference Standard:

1. Goal: There is no goal for RQ, only a reference standard.

   OR

2. Reference standard: A patient/client on parenteral nutrition support with an RQ of 1.04 compared to the reference standard (0.7-1.0) with no apparent errors in the measurement.

Sample monitoring and evaluation documentation

Initial encounter with patient/ client	Patient/client's RQ is 1.04. Will re-measure RQ and rule out measurement error.
Re-assessment after nutrition intervention	No progress toward reference standard as patient/client's RQ is 1.05 with no apparent measurement errors. Will monitor change in RQ after feeding adjustment.

Suggested references for indicators, measurement techniques, and reference standards are available in the International Dietetics and Nutrition Terminology (IDNT) Reference Manual.

SIGN/ SYMPTOM

Edition: 2008

URINE PROFILE (S-2.11)

Definition
Physical and/or chemical properties of urine

Monitoring
Changes in these Potential Indicators:
- Urine color
- Urine osmolality
- Urine specific gravity
- Urine tests (e.g., ketones, sugar, protein)
- Urine volume

Examples of the measurement methods or data sources for these outcome indicators
Observation, biochemical measurement, laboratory report, patient/client report

Typically used to measure the outcomes for the following domains of nutrition interventions
Food and/or nutrient delivery, coordination of nutrition care

Typically used to monitor and evaluate change in the following nutrition diagnoses
Inadequate or excessive fluid intake; inadequate or excessive enteral/parenteral nutrition

Evaluation

Criteria for evaluation
Comparison to Goal or Reference Standard:
1. Goal (tailored to patient/client's needs)
   OR
2. Reference standard

URINE PROFILE (S-2.11)

Patient/Client Example(s)

Example(s) of one or two of the Nutrition Care Indicators for this outcome (*includes sample initial and re-assessment documentation for one of the indicators*)

Indicator(s) selected
Urine specific gravity

Criteria for evaluation
Comparison to Goal or Reference Standard
1. Goal: Not generally used for this indicator.
   OR
2. Reference standard: The patient/client's urine specific gravity is 1.050, which is above* the normal range (using the reference standard of 1.003-1.030).

Sample monitoring and evaluation documentation

Initial encounter with patient/client	Patient/client's urine specific gravity is 1.050, which is above the normal range compared to the reference standard of 1.003-1.030. Will monitor change in urine specific gravity at next encounter.
Re-assessment after nutrition intervention	Significant progress toward goal; patient/client's urine specific gravity is 1.035.

Suggested references for indicators, measurement techniques, and reference standards are available in the International Dietetics and Nutrition Terminology (IDNT) Reference Manual.

*Could be specified as "above," "below," or a "percent of" the reference value.

Edition: 2008

VITAMIN PROFILE (S-2.12)

Definition
Laboratory measures associated with body vitamin status

Monitoring
Changes in these Potential Indicators:
- Vitamin A, serum or plasma retinol
- Vitamin C, plasma or serum
- Vitamin D (25-Hydroxy)
- Vitamin E (plasma alpha-tocopherol)
- Thiamin (activity coefficient for erythrocyte transketolase activity)
- Riboflavin (activity coefficient for erythrocyte glutathione reductase activity)
- Niacin (urinary N'methyl-nicotinamide concentration)
- Vitamin B6 (plasma or serum pyridoxal 5'phosphate) concentration

NOTE: Measures for folate and Vitamin B12 can be found on the Nutritional Anemia Profile reference sheet. Measures related to Vitamin K (PT, PTT, INR) can be found on the GI Profile reference sheet.

Examples of the measurement methods or data sources for these outcome indicators
Biochemical measurement, patient/client record

Typically used to measure the outcomes for the following domains of nutrition interventions
Food and/or nutrient delivery, coordination of nutrition care

Typically used to monitor and evaluate change in the following nutrition diagnoses
Excess or inadequate intake of vitamins

VITAMIN PROFILE (S-2.12)

Evaluation

Criteria for evaluation
Comparison to Goal or Reference Standard:
1. Goal (tailored to patient/client's needs)
OR
2. Reference standard

Patient/Client Example(s)
Example(s) of one or two of the Nutrition Care Indicators for this outcome (*includes sample initial and re-assessment documentation for one of the indicators*)

Indicator(s) selected
Serum retinol

Criteria for evaluation
Comparison to Goal or Reference Standard:
1. Goal: Not generally used for this indicator.
OR
2. Reference standard: The patient/client's serum retinol is 95 μg/dL which is above* the reference standard (10-60 μg/dL).

Sample monitoring and evaluation documentation

Initial encounter with patient/ client	Patient/client's serum retinol is 95 μg/dL. Will monitor change in serum retinol at next encounter.
Re-assessment at a later date	Significant progress toward reference standard. Patient/ client's retinol is 70 μg/dL.

Suggested references for indicators, measurement techniques, and reference standards are available in the International Dietetics and Nutrition Terminology (IDNT) Reference Manual.

*Could be specified as "above," "below," or a "percent of" the reference value.

SIGN/ SYMPTOM

Edition: 2008

NUTRITION PHYSICAL EXAM FINDINGS (S-3.1)

Definition

Nutrition-related physical characteristics associated with pathophysiological states derived from observation or the medical record

Monitoring

Changes in these Potential Indicators:

- Cardiovascular-pulmonary system
    - o   edema, pulmonary (crackles or rales)
- Extremities and musculo-skeletal system
    - o   bones, obvious prominence
    - o   hands/feet, tingling and numbness
    - o   muscle soreness
    - o   nail beds, blue, clubbing, pale
    - o   muscle wasting, subcutaneous fat loss
    - o   excessive subcutaneous fat
    - o   Russell's sign
- Gastrointestinal system
    - o   ascites
    - o   appetite, satiety
    - o   bowel function
    - o   bowel sounds
    - o   distension, abdominal
    - o   gastric residual volume (GRV)
    - o   nausea
    - o   taste alterations
    - o   vomiting
- Head and neck
    Eyes:
    - o   bitot's spots
    - o   night blindness
    - o   xerophthalmia

    Tongue:
    - o   bright red or magenta
    - o   dry or cracked
    - o   glossitis

    Mouth and throat:
    - o   cheilosis
    - o   dry mucus membranes
    - o   gums, inflamed or bleeding
    - o   ketone smell on breath
    - o   lesions, oral
    - o   lips, dry or cracked
    - o   mucosa, edema
    - o   stomatitis

SIGN/
SYMPTOM

NUTRITION PHYSICAL EXAM FINDINGS (S-3.1)

Head:
- o   hair, brittle, lifeless, coiled, or loss
- o   headache
- o   lanugo hair formation
- o   mucosa, dry nasal
- o   temporal wasting

• Neurological system
- o   confusion, concentration
- o   cranial nerve evaluation
- o   motor, fine disturbance
- o   motor, gross and/or gait disturbance
- o   vibratory and position sense

• Skin
- o   acanthanosis nigricans
- o   edema, peripheral
- o   erythema, scaling and peeling
- o   ecchymosis
- o   follicular hyperkeratosis
- o   integrity, turgor
- o   seborrheic dermatitis
- o   perifolicular hemorrhages
- o   petechiae
- o   pressure ulcers (stage II-IV)
- o   wound healing
- o   xanthomas

• Vital signs
- o   blood pressure
- o   respiratory rate

Examples of the measurement methods or data sources for these outcome indicators
Direct observation, patient/client report, medical record

Typically used to measure the outcomes for the following domains of nutrition interventions
Nutrition education, nutrition counseling

Typically used to monitor and evaluate change in the following nutrition diagnoses
Excess or inadequate intake of sodium, vitamins/minerals, fluid, parenteral/enteral nutrition; overweight/obesity

SIGN/
SYMPTOM

NUTRITION PHYSICAL EXAM FINDINGS CONT'D (S-3.1)

Evaluation

Criteria for evaluation

Comparison to Goal or Reference Standard:

1. Goal (tailored to patient/client's needs)

OR

2. Reference standard

Patient/Client Example(s)

Example(s) of one or two of the Nutrition Care Indicators for this outcome (*includes sample initial and re-assessment documentation for one of the indicators*)

Indicator(s) selected

Blood pressure

Criteria for evaluation

Comparison to Goal or Reference Standard:

1. Goal: The patient/client has reduced blood pressure to goal of 135/85 mmHg with weight loss.

OR

2. Reference standard: The patient/client's blood pressure is 150/90 mmHg which is above* the reference standard (< 120/80 mmHg), indicating stage I hypertension.

Sample monitoring and evaluation documentation

Initial encounter with patient/ client	Patient/client's blood pressure is 150/90 mmHg, stage I hypertension. Will monitor change in blood pressure at next encounter.
Re-assessment after nutrition intervention	Significant progress toward reference standard. Patient/ client's blood pressure is 135/82 mmHg.

Suggested references for indicators, measurement techniques, and reference standards are available in the International Dietetics and Nutrition Terminology (IDNT) Reference Manual.

*Could be specified as "above," "below," or a "percent of" the reference value.

SIGN/
SYMPTOM

NUTRITION QUALITY OF LIFE (PC-1.1)

Definition
Extent to which the nutrition care process impacts a patient/client's physical, mental and social well-being related to food and nutrition

Monitoring
Changes in these Potential Indicators:
- Food impact (e.g., choice, available, enjoyable)
- Physical state (e.g., food-related condition impacted activity, sleep, breathing)
- Psychological factors (e.g., positive/negative feelings related to food)
- Self-image
- Self-efficacy (e.g., know what, how much to eat)
- Social/interpersonal factors
- Nutrition quality of life score

NOTE: A nutrition quality of life instrument has been developed and is being validated (Barr JT, et al 2003). Focused questioning around the six indicators using the 50 NQOL statements is recommended. Self-efficacy can be found on the Beliefs and Attitudes Reference Sheet. Social/interpersonal factors can be found Social Support Reference Sheet. Food impact may entail monitoring certain aspects on the Access to Food Reference Sheet. Physical state may entail monitoring physical activity using the Physical Activity Reference Sheet.

Examples of the measurement methods or data sources for these outcome indicators
Nutrition Quality of Life measurement tool, other quality of life tools

Typically used to monitor and evaluate change in the following domains of nutrition interventions
Food and/or nutrient delivery, supplements, nutrition education, nutrition counseling, coordination of nutrition care

Typically used to monitor and evaluate change in the following nutrition diagnoses
Poor nutrition quality of life, inadequate or excessive energy or macronutrient intake, underweight, involuntary weight loss, overweight/obesity, involuntary weight gain, disordered eating pattern, inability or lack of desire to manage self-care, swallowing difficulty, chewing difficulty, self-feeding difficulty, altered GI function, limited access to food

PT CENTERED

Edition: 2008

NUTRITION QUALITY OF LIFE CONT'D (PC-1.1)

Evaluation

Criteria for evaluation
Comparison to Goal or Reference Standard:
1. Goal (tailored to patient/client's needs)
   OR
2. Reference standard

Patient/Client Example(s)
Example(s) of one or two of the Nutrition Care Indicators for this outcome (*includes sample initial and re-assessment documentation for one of the indicators*)

Indicator(s) selected
Nutrition quality of life score

Criteria for evaluation
Comparison to Goal or Reference Standard:
1. Goal: Patient/client with chronic renal disease currently reports poor nutrition quality of life, especially decreased walking ability (physical) and limited food choices on renal diet (food impact). The goal of medical nutrition therapy is to educate and coach patient and his family on options and strategies to significantly enhance his nutrition quality of life.
   OR
2. Reference standard: No validated standard exists.

Sample monitoring and evaluation documentation

Initial encounter with patient/ client	Patient/client with chronic renal disease reports poor nutrition quality of life, particularly in physical and food impact aspects. Patient/client to receive intensive medical nutrition therapy with a goal to improve client's overall nutrition quality of life over a 6-month period. Will monitor nutrition quality of life in 6 months.
Re-assessment after nutrition intervention	Some progress toward goal. Patient/client's nutrition quality of life is increased, but further improvement is desired in the physical dimension. Will continue medical nutrition therapy and reassess in 3 months.

Suggested references for indicators, measurement techniques, and reference standards are available in the International Dietetics and Nutrition Terminology (IDNT) Reference Manual.

PT CENTERED

Terminology Index

Edition: 2008

Edition: 2008

244